THE ONE-POT WEIGHT LOSS PLAN

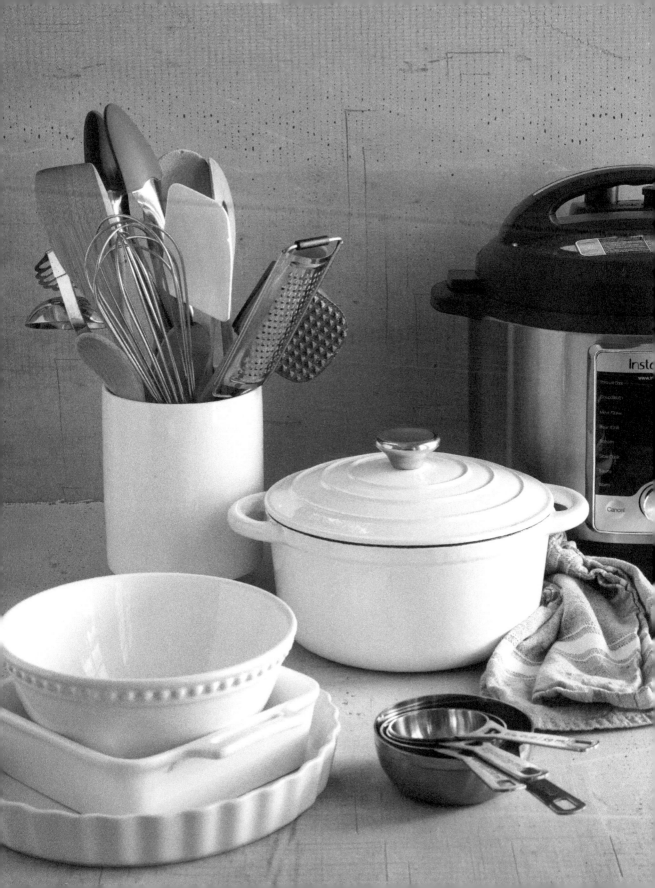

THE ONE-POT
Weight Loss Plan

HEALTHY MEALS FOR YOUR SLOW COOKER, SKILLET, SHEET PAN, AND MORE

SHELLEY RAEL, MS, RDN

ROCKRIDGE
PRESS

———————— ⚓ ————————

FOR THOSE WHO SAY, *"I don't cook."*

IF YOU'D GIVEN UP THE FIRST TIME YOU DIDN'T SUCCEED,

YOU WOULDN'T BE WALKING TODAY.

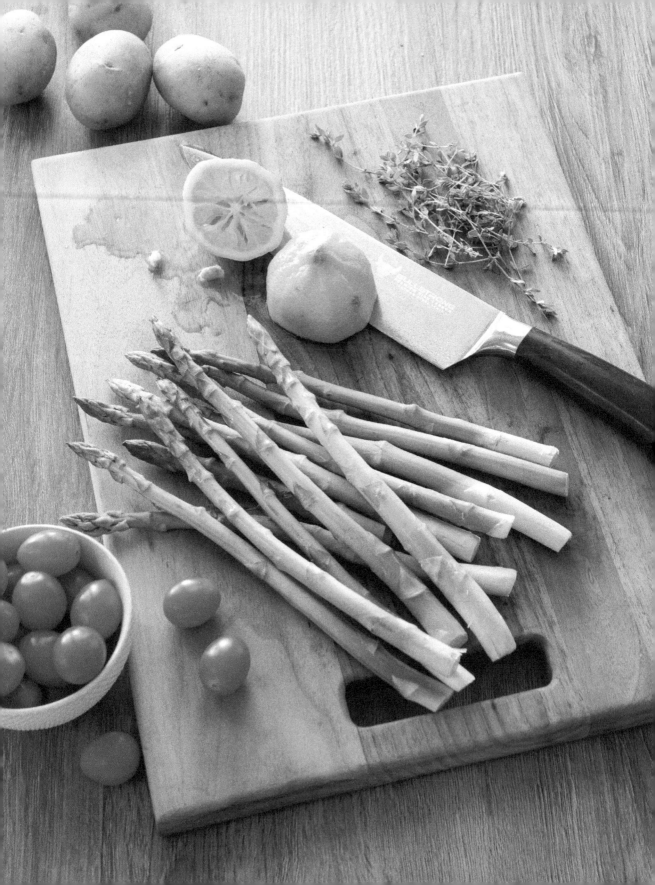

CONTENTS

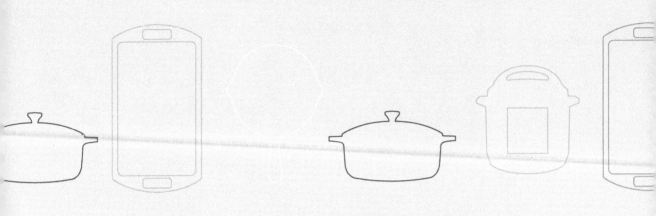

INTRODUCTION

WELCOME TO *The One-Pot Weight Loss Plan.* As a dietitian, I've spent the past twenty years helping people just like you lose weight for good by teaching them how to make healthier food choices. I've worked with people who were not only striving to lose weight, but also improving their health or managing a disease. And I know it isn't easy. Many people have told me that their biggest challenge is that they either don't know what to eat or they don't know how to cook delicious, healthy food quickly and easily. After all, life is busy, and our daily demands only grow each day.

This is why I like the one-pot approach. By reducing the amount of time you spend in the kitchen (with both preparation and cleanup), you'll naturally be more inclined to continue to cook at home. It also empowers you to take control of your health by choosing both the ingredients and portions you're putting into your body. Over the years, I've found that once portion sizes are aligned with your body's needs, the weight comes off naturally.

So here's the good news: Instead of starving yourself or overly restricting your favorite foods, you simply need to focus on eating more appropriate portions for your body. And here's the great news: No food is off-limits. You just choose the foods you *should* have first, then enjoy the foods you *want* to have afterward.

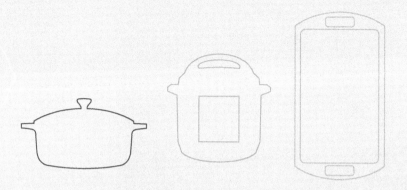
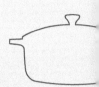

The 28-day plan in this book will set you up for success by showing you several ways to make healthy meals in just minutes each day. After you complete the 28-day plan, you'll have a slew of new healthy habits you can use for life. Once you have the hang of it, you can add new recipes to your weekly menu and continue with your weight loss journey. And while you can dine out on occasion, you'll look and feel so great that you'll actually want to continue making most of your meals at home.

One last piece of advice before you get started: Try to incorporate some exercise. While changing your eating habits is the biggest factor in achieving weight loss, exercise has been shown to enhance your results and makes for a healthier body in general. If you're new to exercise or just haven't done it in a while, don't worry. I'll provide some suggestions in Chapter 2 to get you started.

Congratulations on starting this new chapter in your life and deciding that you're ready to lose weight for good! This plan is so attainable and these recipes are so easy and delicious that you're actually going to look forward to mealtime. And get your family in on the fun, too. Invite them into the kitchen to help with preparation and get excited about what you're all having for dinner tonight. I can't wait to see you on the other side!

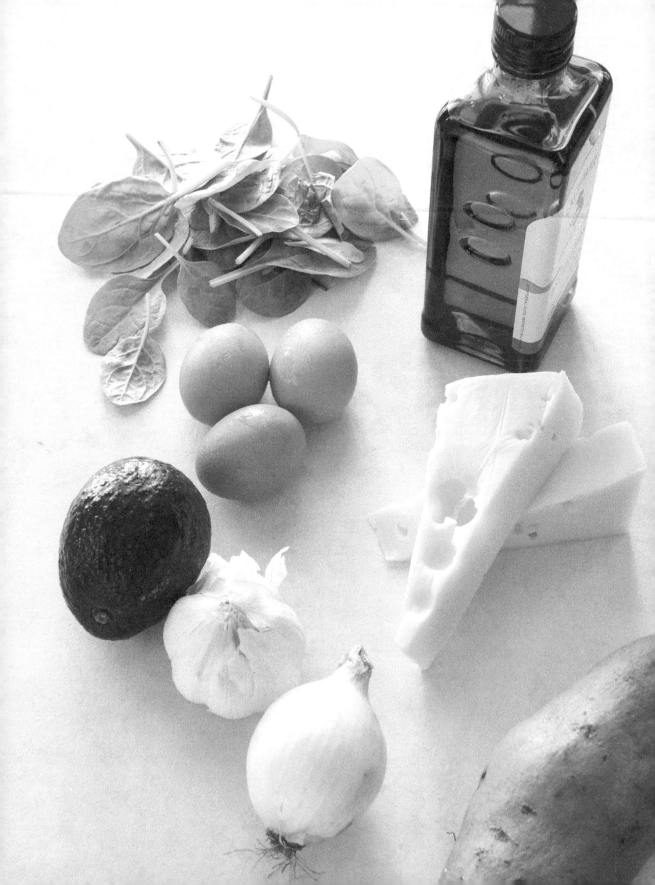

PART ONE

THE DIET *and* MEAL PLAN

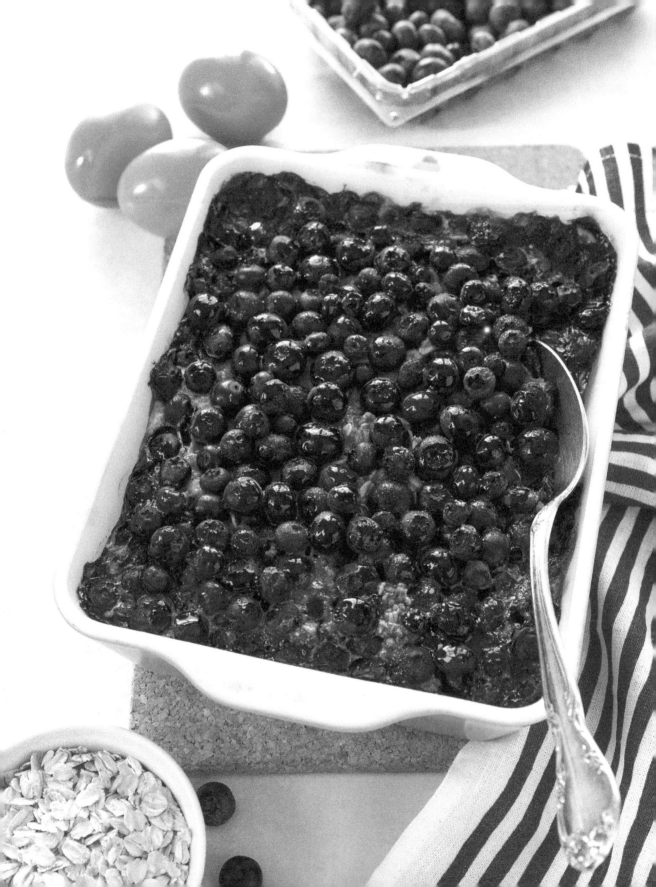

THE ONE-POT WEIGHT LOSS SOLUTION

CONGRATULATIONS ON TAKING THIS STEP IN MAKING a positive lifestyle change! Whether you want to look better, feel healthier, have more energy, or achieve all of these goals, you are already on your way simply by picking up this book. And whether you are doing this with your partner, spouse, family, friends, or by yourself, this book will help you reach your goals.

The information, tips, and 28-day plan in *The One-Pot Weight Loss Plan* will help you make sustainable, lifelong changes. The information here is based on solid, scientifically backed evidence. By adopting the tips in this book, including conscious eating, preparing and cooking healthier versions of your favorite one-pot dishes, and choosing appropriate portions, weight loss will feel effortless.

YOUR WEIGHT LOSS JOURNEY

When people want to lose weight, a "diet" or restriction mind-set frequently comes to mind. Thinking of lists of "off-limits" foods and "I can't eat that" are common in weight loss programs, but that is not real life. Highly restrictive diets help people quickly reach weight loss goals, but once they stop the diet, the weight often returns (and then some).

The One-Pot Weight Loss Plan encourages you to take small steps to reach your goal in a healthy and sustainable way, without feeling deprived of what you want to eat. By making adjustments to ingredients and portion sizes, and by balancing the nutrients you need, you'll eat real, delicious food that everyone in your household will love. As a

Mixed Berry
Crisp, p. 150

bonus, all of the recipes in this book include easily accessible ingredients that you can get at any grocery store. No specialty stores required.

These recipes provide you with an easy way to eat healthier, manage your caloric intake, and control your portions. And because each recipe uses only one cooking vessel, you'll get in and out of the kitchen quickly. There is less to clean up, which means you'll have less mess and less stress. Soon you'll be on your way to sustainable, manageable weight loss.

AVOIDING PROCESSED FOODS

All food is processed to some extent. Harvesting a vegetable is a form of processing. In the context of this book, though, the term "processed food" refers to a food that is often high in calories and added sugars, fats, or sodium but low in nutrients such as fiber, vitamins, and minerals. Processed foods may have vitamins and minerals added back in to boost the nutrients that were removed during processing.

It's important to note that processed foods often have long lists of unfamiliar ingredients. Minimally processed foods have very few ingredients and should be recognizable. For example, prewashed spinach, precooked brown rice, canned beans, or frozen berries will have one or two ingredients, all of which will be familiar to you.

Sometimes it is easy to spot processed foods, such as soda or candy. These contain calories and added sugars but have little to no nutritional value. But processed foods can often be disguised as healthy foods. Here are a few examples.

Reduced-fat peanut butter, low-fat or fat-free baked goods, and reduced-fat salad dressings. In many cases, when compared to their "regular" versions, these low-fat options have the same or similar calories per serving, fewer healthier fats, and more sodium and added sugar.

"Naturally" cured or uncured bacon. Despite what a label may claim, all bacon is cured and has nitrites, just from different sources (often through the use of celery derivatives).

Ready-to-eat cereal "made with whole grains." Having this note doesn't make the cereal a whole-grain product. Instead, it just means whole grain is included somewhere in the ingredients.

"Veggie" chips. In short, these are still chips, which means they're still low in nutrients.

Not a Fad Diet

This is not a fad diet. Fad diets promote a quick fix, involve "magical" foods or food combinations, have strict rules or lists of off-limits foods, and will often recommend cutting out entire food groups or nutrients, such as carbohydrates. While most of these diets do result in fast weight loss, that success is almost always temporary.

A healthy diet that promotes weight loss must have a balance of macronutrients (carbohydrates, protein, and dietary fat) and create a calorie deficit while still providing the nutrients you need so that you can feel good, use a realistic approach, and include delicious, healthy meals.

The recipes here are versatile and flavorful yet easy and familiar. They include widely available vegetables, whole grains, and both plant- and animal-based proteins. If you have any dietary restrictions, you'll find that all of these recipes will work with minor substitutions.

Busy *and* Healthy

Many times, people think that eating healthily takes a lot of time. Everyone is busy with work, family, and social obligations, but a hectic schedule does not have to come at the expense of eating healthy foods. This book helps you prepare healthy meals quickly, with less equipment and less mess. You *can* live a healthy life while being busy and on the go. You just need to learn the simple steps for living a healthy lifestyle.

WHOLE FOODS

The term "whole foods" is used a lot, but not everyone understands what it means. It is referring not to a specific place to shop but to the overarching approach to food choices. Whole foods are minimally processed and unrefined foods, so you'll usually find them in the produce, dairy, and butcher sections of your local grocery store. These foods include fruits and vegetables, milk, meats, beans, nuts, and whole grains such as oats, brown rice, and quinoa. You can also find them in the frozen foods and canned goods sections, if you know what to look for.

For example, you can buy precooked brown rice in the packaged food or frozen food aisles. A glance at the ingredients list will reveal two things: brown rice and water. Some foods will have several ingredients listed; that doesn't mean they must be avoided, but be aware of the difference. For example, plain yogurt has only a few ingredients, but

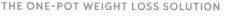

flavored yogurt will have a longer list you must read through. Here's another common example: Regular potato or corn chips have only three ingredients, but that doesn't make it a healthier chip. Avoid foods with hydrogenated or partially hydrogenated oil in the ingredients list. Ingredients are listed in order of quantity, so the first ingredient is the main ingredient in the food.

It's important to note that processed foods are not considered whole foods. Examples of processed foods are packaged foods such as cookies, chips, bacon, deli meats, ready-to-eat cereal, and many energy or protein bars.

Why Eat Whole Foods?

By focusing on whole foods, you know what you are putting into your body. There are no confusing ingredients, no hidden calories, no added sugars, and no added fats. This is a great solution for busy people because figuring out what's in processed foods can take a lot of time and effort.

According to the World Health Organization, there is also a link between processed foods (which are often high in calories, added sugar, added sodium, and added fats) and diseases, including certain cancers, type 2 diabetes, heart disease, and stroke. Eating healthier doesn't guarantee you'll be disease free, but integrating more whole foods into your diet and cutting down on processed foods can significantly decrease the risk.

Excessive red- and processed-meat consumption is associated with heart disease, stroke, type 2 diabetes, obesity, and some cancers. It is important to note that meat consumption alone is not the cause of diseases, but high red-meat intake is indicative of the overall pattern of unhealthy eating. In fact, according to a study in the journal *Public Health Nutrition*, if people increased their consumption of plant-based foods, they could reduce their risk of each of the previously mentioned diseases.

Accordingly, *The One-Pot Weight Loss Plan* includes a variety of recipes that primarily use whole foods and minimize meat consumption. Each chapter contains vegetarian or pescatarian options, and most recipes with meat include meatless alternatives.

The Research

The recipes in this book are optimized for complex carbs, healthy fats, and lean proteins because research shows that these foods promote weight loss and help prevent disease.

Complex carbohydrates, such as those in beans, whole grains, and vegetables, are also rich in fiber. Consuming fiber-rich foods, which are high in nutrients and often contain fewer calories than lower-fiber foods, promotes weight loss by suppressing hunger and promoting satiety (or giving a feeling of fullness). As described in the book *Eat for Life: The Food and Nutrition Board's Guide to Reducing Your Risk of Chronic Disease*, integrating these fiber-rich complex carbohydrates into your diet also reduces the risk of diabetes, heart disease, and certain cancers.

Healthy fats, including monounsaturated fatty acids and polyunsaturated fatty acids, are found in fatty fish, nuts, olive oil, and avocados. Eating healthy fats (not low-fat food) helps reduce the risk of heart disease and certain cancers. It also aids weight loss by providing flavor and increasing satiety, which can decrease overall calories consumed.

Lean protein eaten throughout the day, not just with dinner, also helps you feel fuller longer, leading you to eat less and lose more weight. Lean protein includes both animal and plant sources. Fish and shellfish, chicken and turkey, and lean beef and pork provide lean protein, as do beans and lentils, low-fat dairy such as Greek yogurt and cottage cheese, and tofu. Integrating more plant-based protein sources can reduce the risk of chronic diseases because they contribute additional disease-fighting nutrients.

The best way to integrate high-fiber complex carbohydrates, healthy fats, and lean protein is to choose whole foods and minimally processed foods. Processed foods tend to be low in complex carbohydrates and high in unhealthy fats.

Whole Foods + One Pot

Combining a whole-foods diet with a one-pot strategy will help simplify cooking and eating for you. When you choose whole foods, you know exactly what you need and what you are using in the recipes. There's no guesswork about what's going into your food. The one-pot strategy means you don't need multiple pots and pans or appliances to make each meal, making it easier—and more enjoyable—to sustain healthy cooking. Plus, these one-pot recipes are designed with flavor in mind. The idea is simple: If food tastes good and is easy to prepare, you'll be more likely to continue cooking and eating healthier.

Here's a list of simple healthy swaps you can try to get a head start. It'll also help you to adapt some of your current favorite dishes to be weight loss–friendly!

INSTEAD OF . . .	TRY . . .	BECAUSE . . .
Brown Sugar	Maple Syrup	Pure maple syrup provides less sweetener and more vitamins and minerals. Use 3 tablespoons pure maple syrup in place of 4 tablespoons brown sugar.
Butter	Avocado	Avocado provides fewer calories, less total fat and saturated fat, and more vitamins and minerals.
Butter	Olive Oil	These have the same calorie and fat content, but olive oil has a healthier fat profile.
Ground Meat (beef or turkey)	Mushrooms	Mushrooms contribute a meaty texture and have only 15 calories per cup. They also add vitamins and minerals. Mushrooms can expand or replace meat for a lower-calorie option.
Iceberg Lettuce	Spinach or Kale	Both spinach and kale have more vitamins and minerals than iceberg lettuce.
Potatoes	Cauliflower	Cauliflower is lower in calories; substitute it for all or part of your mashed or roasted potatoes to cut calories and add nutrients.
Rice	Riced Cauliflower	This substitution cuts calories and adds nutrients.
Salt	Herb and Spice Blends	The blend of herbs and spices boosts flavor and contains less sodium.
Sour Cream	Plain, Fat-Free Greek Yogurt	Greek yogurt contains fewer calories, less fat, and more protein than sour cream.
Spaghetti (made from wheat)	Spaghetti Squash	Spaghetti squash is lower in calories and higher in vitamins and minerals than traditional spaghetti.
Sugar	Ripe Bananas	This substitution increases vitamins and minerals in smoothies, baked goods, and frozen desserts. Remember, the riper the banana, the sweeter the taste.
White Wine	Broth	Broth is nonalcoholic and contains fewer calories than white wine.

Canned and Frozen Foods

Having fresh fruits and vegetables is great, but it's not always realistic. You may be surprised to learn that frozen and canned fruits and vegetables are often just as healthy, and they can save both time and money and reduce food waste.

When choosing frozen foods, make sure that the only ingredients listed are water and the item you are buying. For instance, frozen broccoli should contain only broccoli and water.

When choosing canned vegetables and beans, choose low-sodium options whenever possible, and make sure to drain and rinse them as part of preparation. This will help reduce the overall sodium content.

When choosing canned fruit, choose fruit "in its own juice" whenever possible. Avoid the heavy and light syrup options so that you aren't consuming added sugars.

When choosing precooked grains such as brown rice or quinoa, be sure that the grain and water are the only ingredients.

There's no need to avoid frozen or canned fruits, vegetables, beans, and fish. Having them on hand will save you some prep time and ensure that you have ingredients ready for last-minute meals.

Should I Buy Organic?

A common misperception is that organic food is more nutritious than conventionally grown food. If you prefer organic foods, and they fit in your budget, buy them. But, to date, there is no evidence that organic foods have different nutritional values. Regardless of the type of fruits and vegetables you buy, always wash them with water before slicing, peeling, or eating. This will wash away any residues left from the growing process or the fingers of anyone who handled it between the harvest and your home. You may see lists that suggest the top dozen foods to always buy organic and the foods you don't need to worry about. You can skip these lists; even foods with a "high" pesticide residue are still far below what is considered acceptable. According to the pesticide residue calculator at www.safefruitsandveggies.com, a person would likely have to eat several servings of that food on a daily basis to even come close to an unsafe level. It's better to eat any kind of fruits and vegetables rather than skip them because they are not organic.

Cooking at home is a great way to keep costs down, manage portions, and have control over what goes into your meals. Remember that foods high in fiber and lean protein will help you feel full and stay satisfied. And here's another bonus: When you base your meals around filling fruits, vegetables, whole grains, and lean protein, you can also save money by eating less.

Here are three tips to help you keep costs down as you shop and plan your weekly meals:

Cook once, serve twice. Tonight's dinner can also be tomorrow's lunch. You may need to double the recipe or just portion out the appropriate number of servings from the original recipe, but this strategy saves you the cost (and the calories) of going out for lunch.

Shop your kitchen. Use ingredients you already have in your pantry, freezer, or refrigerator. If you don't need more, don't buy them. Substitute an ingredient for something you already have, such as spinach instead of kale or green beans instead of broccoli.

Plan ahead. Outline what meals you will make this week and be sure that you'll have time in your schedule that day to cook. Review the ingredients and note what groceries you need, comparing them to what you already have in your kitchen. If you are motivated, do some prep over the weekend, such as chopping vegetables for the week ahead to save time later. By planning ahead, you'll be less likely to dine out on a whim, which will help you save some money.

Substitutions

The ingredients in these recipes should be available in your local grocery store. If you're shopping seasonally, use food of similar taste and texture (for instance, substitute spinach for Swiss chard). If you don't have access to a vegetable the recipe calls for, or if you don't care for it, find an alternative that suits your preference rather than skipping it altogether. For example, if you don't like asparagus, use fresh green beans. If you don't like beets, use sweet potatoes or butternut squash. Many recipes will include suggestions for suitable substitutions, and you can experiment to find what you like.

NAVIGATING THE GROCERY STORE

When you're shopping, prioritize these sections: fresh produce, butcher, refrigerator, freezer, and the aisles with canned fruits and vegetables, canned beans, dried grains and beans, spices, vinegars, and oils. The best way to avoid processed foods such as ready-to-eat cereals, snack foods, bottled drinks, baked goods, processed deli meats, and heat-and-serve meals is to not have them in the house, so skip those aisles in the grocery store.

Here are some tips for grocery shopping for weight loss:

Make a list. To avoid forgetting the list at home, put the list directly into your Notes app or another app on your phone.

Stick to the list. Only go down the aisles pertaining to your list, which will help you avoid impulse buys.

Don't shop hungry. Hunger can lead to impulse purchases and choosing unhealthy foods.

Shop without the kids. It may not always be practical or possible, but when you can, focusing on what you need rather than what they want will save you both money and stress.

Use grocery pickup or delivery. Many stores now offer curbside pickup at no additional charge. Simply order your items on the store's app, choose your pickup time, and get exactly what you need without wandering the aisles and the checkout line.

BALANCING YOUR MACROS

The term "macros" refers to macronutrients, the nutrients humans need in large amounts. Nutrients fall into six categories: carbohydrates, fat, protein, vitamins, minerals, and water. Calories come directly from carbohydrates, fat, and protein, which are considered macronutrients because humans need them in larger amounts. Conversely, vitamins and minerals are known as micronutrients and are needed in smaller amounts.

Most food has a variety of all the nutrients, but no single food has all the nutrients the human body needs. As a result, it can be confusing to call a single food a carbohydrate or a protein. For example, carbohydrates are in all plant foods and dairy products. Likewise, protein is found in all food in varying amounts. Fats are also found in a variety of foods, but many foods are naturally fat-free. All whole foods and minimally processed foods will have a combination of at least two macronutrients, and they often contain all three.

In general, people should aim for an overall diet that provides 45 percent of their calories from carbohydrates, 30 percent from fat, and 25 percent from protein. This is a general, flexible guideline, meaning that not every food, meal, or even daily intake will result in these exact percentages, but it averages out. Individual needs vary, so this is just a starting point to help you find what works for your body's needs.

An abundance of research, along with recommendations from organizations such as the American Cancer Society, American Diabetes Association, and American Heart Association, recommends reducing added sugars and refined grains, which are stripped of their naturally occurring nutrients, and increasing complex carbohydrates such as whole grains and high-fiber fruits and vegetables.

Lean protein sources are also recommended. These include quinoa, beans, seafood such as fish and shellfish, poultry such as chicken and turkey, and lean cuts of red meats that include the terms "round," "loin," or "sirloin" in the name.

There are several types of fats: saturated, monounsaturated, and polyunsaturated. Minimize saturated fats that are solid at room temperature, including most animal fats, butter, and coconut oil. Monounsaturated fat is a healthier fat and is found in avocados, olive oil, and most nuts and seeds. Polyunsaturated fat is also healthier and is found in walnuts, soybeans, and fatty fish, including salmon and tuna.

The key to following a healthy diet that supports weight loss is not choosing lower fat overall, but choosing more unsaturated fats and less saturated fat, which helps reduce the risk of chronic diseases.

Calories in, Calories Out

To achieve weight loss, a calorie deficit is essential. This means that you must take in fewer calories than your body uses on a daily basis.

So, if you use 2,000 calories per day and you're taking in 2,000 calories per day, your weight will remain stable. Conversely, if you use 2,000 calories per day but take in 1,600 calories per day, you will be in a calorie deficit but still getting all the nutrients you need.

The meal plan in this book is designed for a 1,600-calorie diet. Because *The One-Pot Weight Loss Plan* is written for a variety of readers, you can adjust your calories up or down, depending on where you are starting from.

Integrating exercise will also help create a calorie deficit. For more on incorporating regular exercise, see page 27.

YOUR MACRO BREAKDOWN

The breakdown of the 1,600 calories recommended in this meal plan is as follows:

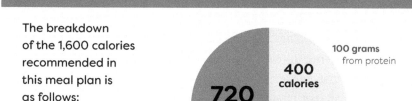

400 calories   100 grams from protein

720 calories

180 grams total carbohydrates

480 calories   53 grams of total fat

Note: Choose whole-food complex carbohydrates to get at least 25 grams of fiber and less than 25 grams from added sugars.

Portion Size

One of the easiest ways to control calories, eat what you want, and still lose weight is to manage your portion sizes. With one-pot recipes, it's easy to divide the entire meal into its respective portions without having to calculate various side dishes and sauces.

The one-pot method means the entire meal is a single dish. When a recipe states that it "serves 4," make sure the recipe is served in four evenly divided portions. When it's time to serve the meal, portion out all the servings immediately. For example, if tonight's meal serves four and there are two people eating, then serve out two plates or bowls and use two reusable storage containers right away for the rest, ensuring the four servings remain intact.

Why are portions so important? If a recipe serves four and has 350 calories per serving (1,400 calories in the entire dish), and that very same recipe is divided into three servings instead, then each serving will have 467 calories, over 100 more calories than it's supposed to! Those extra calories add up and may stall your weight loss.

Exercise

In the discussion of a healthy lifestyle, it is impossible to exclude exercise. According to a review published in the *Canadian Medical Association Journal,* there are numerous benefits to regular exercise. Burning calories to enhance weight loss is one benefit, but exercise is also known to reduce the risk of several chronic diseases and help manage existing health conditions. Regular exercise may reduce your risk of heart disease and improve blood pressure and cholesterol levels; regulate blood sugar and insulin levels, which helps manage or reduce your risk for type 2 diabetes; strengthen bones and muscles; and even reduce the risk of certain cancers. The immediate impact is that it gives you more energy, helps you sleep better, decreases stress, and improves your mood. You will find more information on how to start an accessible, beginner-level exercise program in Chapter 2.

The best exercise is one you enjoy and will do at your convenience. Some people want to exercise first thing in the morning, while others will take part of their lunch break to exercise. If you aren't a morning person or your lunch break isn't convenient, then find a time that does work for you. If you are intimidated by a gym, then do routines at home. Another great tip is to recruit an exercise buddy for accountability. Even if you don't exercise together, you can check in with each other. By keeping it simple, you'll work your way into a new regular routine.

ONE-POT WEIGHT LOSS

One-pot meals work well for weight loss for a variety of reasons. As we've discussed, because they can be easily divided, they support portion control. The cooking methods also reduce the need for added fats, which quickly add unnecessary calories.

This type of cooking is also designed with your busy lifestyle in mind; one-pot meals provide enough food for the whole family to enjoy, set you up with leftovers, and make weekday meal prep and cleanup quicker and simpler. All of these factors mean you'll be more likely to stick to the plan.

Most important, the recipes are varied, delicious, and easy, making this a sustainable way to eat, not just another temporary diet. These one-pot meals set you up for weight loss success for life.

YOUR ONE-POT KITCHEN

All the recipes in this book are made in a single small appliance, pot, pan, or dish. Each chapter has recipes using just that pot, including breakfasts, main meals, and desserts.

Electric Pressure Cooker

Electric pressure cookers have become popular in recent years. Today's pressure cookers are safer than the stovetop cookers of the past. Because they shorten the cooking time of most meals by at least half and there is no need to constantly monitor them as the food cooks, they are convenient kitchen countertop appliances.

Some electric pressure cookers may multitask as a slow cooker, steamer, and even a sauté pan. This can help reduce the number of appliances in your kitchen. Most have digital readouts and a variety of settings, and are programmable to delay the start time. Some are even capable of being programmed remotely. The price will vary based on the number of features. Find one that best suits your needs and has the features you want. (A 6-quart stainless steel model should meet the needs of a family of four.)

Many things can be made in a pressure cooker, from hard-boiled eggs to desserts, dried beans to meat, and rice to vegetables. Pressure cookers work through steaming, which is one of the best cooking methods to retain nutrients in foods.

Slow Cooker

There are many types of slow cookers on the market. Some have simple low, medium, and high settings. Others are programmable to both temperature and length of cooking time and allow for a delayed start time. Some are strictly slow cookers while others contain a sauté or browning feature that allows more versatility of recipes and eliminates the need to start a dish in a sauté pan on the stove before moving it to the slow cooker.

Many slow cooker recipes take four to six hours, so a "keep warm" feature that holds the food to temperature while not continuing to cook is helpful if you aren't ready to eat as soon as you walk in the door or when the food is ready.

A popular size is a 6- to 7-quart capacity pot. A removable pot is essential for cleaning, and pots may be stainless steel or ceramic. It's important to note that while durable, a ceramic pot is more prone to damage and is heavier than the stainless-steel versions. A locking lid is necessary only if you plan to travel with the slow cooker.

Cooking foods at lower temperatures for longer periods of time results in greater flavor. More flavor means little to no added fat and salt. The slow cooker is great for cold-weather meals, such as stew and soups, but it also puts out less heat than an oven, so it may be ideal for warmer days as well.

Dutch Oven

A Dutch oven is a larger cooking pot with a lid. It often has two handles and can be transferred from the stovetop to the oven. A Dutch oven can be purchased by itself but is frequently part of a multipiece cookware set.

A traditional Dutch oven is made of cast iron or aluminum, but some are ceramic and may have an enamel coating. A cast-iron Dutch oven is heavy by itself, and the addition of food makes it heavier. With recipes moving from the stovetop to the oven, this is a consideration. While these vessels come in many sizes, the recipes in this book call for a 6-quart Dutch oven, so make sure that's the size you have on hand or pick one up at the store. Also, ensure that all materials, including the lid, are oven-safe up to 500°F.

Dutch ovens can be used for making soups, stews, and stir-fries, cooking meats and fish, and even baking bread. Many recipes will start with browning the foods "dry" (with little to no liquid), then stewing or simmering the food in liquid until it's fully cooked. This may be done on the stovetop or completed in the oven.

Because the Dutch oven allows for many cooking methods, including braising (which minimizes added fat), using one will enhance your flavors and allow for variety.

Blender

There are a variety of blenders on the market. Some are designed for just making smoothies, while others have more versatile uses, like turning nuts into nut butter.

A blender container that has measurements marked on it allows you to measure directly into the container, minimizing the use of additional measuring tools. The material of the blender doesn't matter as much as the capacity. Use at least an 8- to 10-cup capacity blender when making the recipes in this book.

As a general rule, the lower the price of a blender, the lower the speed and power. The good news is that only a few speeds are necessary, unless you plan to make your own nut butter. The recipes in this book work for blenders with just a few speeds and a 500-watt motor.

The blender is best used for smoothies; soups that can be served cold or at room temperature or require reheating; and puddings. Blender-based dishes can be made healthier by integrating a wide variety of fruits and vegetables that you may not normally eat. Adding spinach or kale to a green smoothie or including more vegetables in a puréed soup can easily increase the nutrients in your meals.

Soup Pot

As the name indicates, the soup pot is best for soups and stews. There is a variety of soups and stews that are both balanced and nutritious. In fact, making soups and stews can help you integrate more vegetables and protein into your diet while still retaining a rich flavor.

Soup pots may also be referred to as stockpots. They come with lids, and some even include an insert that can be used as a strainer or steamer. This isn't a necessary component, but it is convenient to have.

Soup pots can serve a similar purpose as a Dutch oven, but a soup pot is not intended to go into the oven—it stays on the cooktop. When it comes to size, compared to a Dutch oven, a soup pot is generally taller.

Stainless steel or aluminum pots are widely available, but for durability and even heating, anodized aluminum is recommended. A 6- to 8-quart capacity soup pot will work perfectly for the recipes in this book. If you plan to double recipes regularly, then use a 10- to 12-quart pot.

Casserole Dish and Sheet Pan

Sheet pans come in various sizes referred to as quarter, half, or full. The most common size used in *The One-Pot Weight Loss Plan* is the half-sheet pan (13-by-18 inches). If you're making smaller batches, you can also use a quarter-sheet pan (9-by-13 inches). Aluminum is the most common material for sheet pans, and you can get them at any big-box store that sells kitchenware or a restaurant supply store.

Sheet pans are best for roasting vegetables, as well as protein such as salmon or chicken. For even quicker cleanup, use parchment paper or aluminum foil to line the sheet pan. Since there is usually little to no additional fat needed, and roasting or caramelizing (the browning of vegetables) elicits lots of flavor, sheet pans provide tasty, effortlessly healthy food.

Casserole dishes can vary widely in sizes, material, and shapes, and they are versatile. Choose ceramic or glass and, ideally, one that comes with a glass lid for use in the oven and a plastic sealable lid for storing leftovers.

Casseroles are assembled in the dish and usually stay in the oven for the entire cooking time, unlike the Dutch oven, which may go from stovetop to oven. In many cases, casseroles may be assembled up to a day in advance and kept covered in the refrigerator until it is time to cook. While this will save on preparation, it will also extend the cooking time to compensate for the colder temperature when you start cooking.

HEALTHY KIDS

Whether you have kids in your household or ones who visit, the meals in this book are intended for the whole family, both adults and children. Many meals are also designed to work as leftovers for tomorrow's lunch, but it may not be reasonable to expect that kids will pack those leftovers for lunch or warm them up on their own. Of course, some meals may be a hit and some may miss. But before assuming anything, have kids try the dishes along with you and let them decide for themselves if they like the dishes or not.

Lunch and snack ideas for kids (and grown-ups, too) include the following:

- "Kebabs" with grapes, strawberries, rotisserie chicken, and cheese cubes on bamboo skewers.

- A sliced fruit-and-nut-butter sandwich, such as almond butter and apples on whole-grain bread or a natural peanut butter and banana "burrito" using a whole wheat tortilla.

- Greek yogurt dip and vegetables such as baby carrots, raw broccoli, snap peas, sliced bell peppers, and cucumbers. Make the dip by mixing together 1 cup plain Greek yogurt, ½ teaspoon onion powder, ½ teaspoon garlic powder, 1 teaspoon dried dill, 1 teaspoon salt, and 1 teaspoon lemon juice.

Salad Bowl

Salad bowls are used for more than just salad. They can be glass, stainless steel, or even ceramic and come in various sizes. While a smaller bowl might be the right size for serving, there may not be enough room to mix and toss the ingredients without making a mess. When in doubt, go up a size.

Recipes using the one-bowl method are usually cold dishes that work well in warmer weather.

Skillet

Skillets are probably one of the first pans people get when setting up a kitchen. You can buy them individually, but multipiece cookware sets usually include two sizes.

Sauté pans also fall into this cooking vessel category. A sauté pan is similar to a skillet, but skillets have slanted sides while sauté pans have straight sides. Often, these two can be used interchangeably. Sauté pans also typically come with lids, while skillets do not. Both will have a single long handle. Larger versions may have a smaller secondary handle on the opposite side to allow for easier movement of the pan.

Cast-iron skillets are versatile and can go from stovetop to oven as needed. In the past, it could take several years to "season" cast iron, giving it a smoother, nonstick cooking surface and preventing rust, but most new versions are already seasoned. Cast iron can still rust, so always dry a cast-iron skillet immediately after washing. Do not let it air-dry.

Iron and aluminum pans are the preferred material for skillets. While copper heats evenly, it is costly and can react with certain types of foods, giving it a metallic taste. Stainless steel is low maintenance, but it doesn't heat evenly. Aluminum heats well but is soft, meaning it can dent easily. Anodized aluminum is treated to make it much more durable and scratch resistant. Iron also heats evenly and is reactive to certain foods, but this is beneficial because it adds iron to your diet without adding the metallic taste that copper gives.

Many skillets are nonstick after a few uses, but even if a skillet is labeled as nonstick, foods can stick if cooked improperly. When choosing a skillet, a 10-inch size is usually appropriate. A 12-inch option may be too large for daily use. An 8-inch skillet is a great size for cooking one or two eggs or making a grilled cheese sandwich, but it's not usually large enough for multiple servings.

Skillets are versatile and can be used to sauté vegetables, brown and cook meats, and even make breakfast foods such as frittatas, pancakes, and French toast. If you want to move a skillet from stovetop to oven, make sure it's oven-safe. Many can go into the oven, but some materials on the handle may not withstand an oven temperature above 400°F.

In many cases, little or even no fat is necessary for nonstick pans. Sautéing vegetables in the skillet lightly cooks them without making them soggy and unappetizing. And remember, good-tasting vegetables always get eaten.

Other Tools

There are many additional kitchen tools and gadgets you may already be using to prep your meals. While there are stores dedicated to kitchen "necessities," many of those items are just "nice to have" gadgets that are unnecessary and serve the same function as a regular knife, spatula, or spoon.

While the recipes in this book don't require much beyond the cooking vessels in each chapter, there are some basic tools that are used over and over and should be part of every kitchen. Here is a quick overview of the basic tools you'll need. You likely already have them in your kitchen.

Chef's Knife

Many knife sets come with a storage block and 8 to 10 knives, including specialty knives that will never be used. Skip the knife sets and purchase an 8- to 10-inch chef's knife instead. While it may seem bigger than you initially need, it will work for most of your cutting needs, from chopping vegetables to slicing meats. Remember that a dull knife is dangerous and may slip, so make sure to keep it sharp with a sharpening steel.

Spring Tongs

Tongs help with both cooking and serving. Spring-loaded handles are nice, and having both a long-handled and short-handled pair will meet most of your needs. There's no need to go fancy. You can get these in most big-box stores for about $10, or visit a restaurant supply store and get a few different sizes.

Bamboo or Wooden Spoons

Whether sautéing, mixing, or tossing, a set of bamboo or other wooden spoons can serve a variety of functions. Bamboo is a sustainable wood that can go in the dishwasher, making cleanup a breeze.

Measuring Cups

Dry measuring cups tend to come in sets of four or more (such as ¼ cup, ⅓ cup, ½ cup, and 1 cup). As the name suggests, these are for dry ingredients such as shredded cheese, cocoa powder, and sugar.

Liquid measuring cups are usually glass or plastic containers that come in 1-cup, 2-cup, and 4-cup sizes. A 2-cup measuring cup will be used most often in the recipes throughout this book to measure liquids such as broth, milk, vinegar, and oil.

Measuring Spoons

You'll use measuring spoons in almost every recipe. Measuring spoon sets will have at least four spoons, but they may have six or more. While they come on a ring, you can remove it. After all, there's no need to pull out the entire set when you're only using a single teaspoon or tablespoon.

THE IMPORTANCE OF MEASURING INGREDIENTS

While you don't need to measure food after it's cooked to track what you eat, measuring ingredients as you make the recipe is crucial for your weight loss success. Measuring the amount of oil you're using rather than just pouring and "eyeballing" it can have a big impact on total calories in the dish and your overall caloric intake. Additionally, when serving, divide the dish into its portions. If a recipe states that it serves four, make sure that there are four servings. Plate all four servings right away, regardless of whether four people are eating or not. Pack extra servings into separate containers.

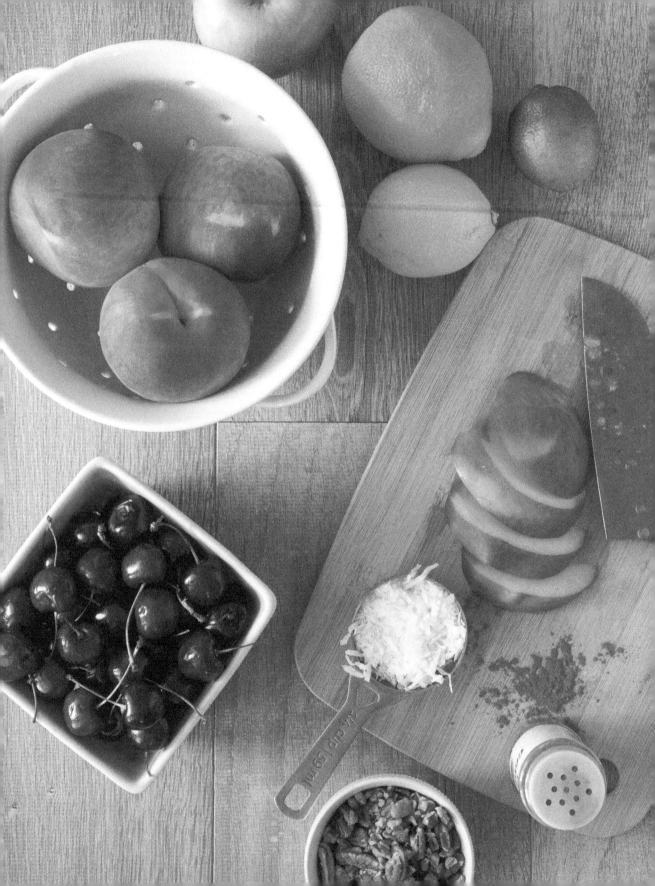

THE 28-DAY MEAL PLAN

HAVING A DETAILED PLAN to follow is critical for success. You can start to exercise more, eat healthier foods, and lose weight without a plan, but it will make your goals much more difficult to achieve. Whether you plan ahead for the full 28 days, want to take it a week at a time, or are just thinking a few days ahead, this plan is a map for your new healthy lifestyle. As you enter the 28-day plan, remember that plans can be flexible, but they should not be ignored. Make sure you always have a backup just in case something comes up at the last minute that interferes with your ability to exercise or prepare that night's meal.

Always remember that this is about progress, not perfection. Look at the meal and exercise plan as a framework, and adjust it to your needs. It is designed to get you going so that you can continue on your own. Set a start date, review the plan in this chapter, customize it as needed to make it yours, and get started!

THE MEAL PLAN

As you read through the meal plan below, set realistic goals and expectations for yourself. Resolve to cook and eat healthy meals for four weeks. This is a doable and flexible plan that accommodates the fluctuations in your daily schedule. Some meals can be assembled, prepped, and even cooked ahead of time, and others don't require any cooking at all.

There are also helpful grocery lists for each week's plan. If they're convenient, use them for your weekly trips to the grocery store, or you can make your own. Some items on the grocery list are staples you already have, and all of them should be readily available at your grocery store for convenient, one-stop shopping.

Meal Prep

Meal prep may vary based on your schedule and preferences. Some people prefer to spend an afternoon over the weekend or at the beginning of the week preparing some of the meals for the coming week. This may include washing and chopping vegetables to save time on the day of the meal, or it may involve cooking in advance so that all you have to do is reheat the food when you're ready to eat it.

Meal prep saves time during the week by cutting down on preparation time the day of the meal. You will be storing the prepped meals in the refrigerator, so make sure you have room.

Here are some tips for meal prep:

Do what works for you. Prepping may include assembling five days of breakfasts or snacks, such as assembling containers for overnight oats without the liquid or getting a week's worth of afternoon snacks ready to take to work.

Take it a few days at a time. If prepping is new to you, consider prepping two or three meals rather than meals for the entire week.

Match your meals to your weekly plans. Plan what you are having for dinner each night in the coming week and what day you are eating it. If you have an evening meeting or after-school sporting events to attend, this may determine which meals to prep earlier in the week.

Get chopping. If the week ahead has recipes that call for cut vegetables such as carrots, celery, onions, or peppers, spend 20 to 30 minutes chopping those and storing them in separate reusable containers. This saves extra time when you're preparing dinner.

Make it a family affair. Use an assembly line method and recruit family members to do their part: adding, cutting, or cooking ingredients.

Pre-portion your servings. Consider making and cooking a casserole or slow cooker meal over the weekend and dividing it into individual containers that can go from freezer or refrigerator to oven or microwave. You'll have an individual serving for each meal ready to go.

Adjustments

The recipes in this book vary in the number of servings, so check this first when planning to make a recipe. Some serve one; others make six or eight servings. The average is four servings. If you have a larger household, you may want to double some recipes. If you have a household of two, this will make the first meal and two leftover servings. If you are cooking for yourself, you can cut some recipes in half, or make the full recipe and divide and freeze portions for the coming weeks.

By making a recipe that serves more than what you need for the first meal, you'll be preparing and cooking meals less often. Having leftovers or additional servings is a good backup plan for unexpected conflicts or when arriving home later than planned.

BEFORE YOU BEGIN

People often get sidetracked from their plans because they have trouble breaking old habits. This section will review the steps you need to take before you start the meal plan to ensure that you have the best chance for success.

Clean Out Your Pantry

Many foods are easy to overconsume because they are designed to create the desire for more. These are highly processed foods with added sugar, fat, and sodium. The easiest way to avoid these foods is to get rid of what you have and make sure you don't buy them going forward.

Remove the following items from your pantry:

- Snack chips
- Soda
- Candy
- Presweetened, ready-to-eat cereal or any cereal that is not a whole grain
- Canned ready-to-eat meals
- Canned meats
- Baking mixes

- Shortening
- Crackers, pastas, and breads that are not whole grain
- Syrups (pure maple syrup is an exception and is used in some of the recipes)
- Peanut butter and nut butter with hydrogenated or partially hydrogenated oils in the ingredients list

Get Enough Sleep

One of the major components of living a healthier lifestyle is getting enough sleep—specifically, enough quality sleep. While you're sleeping, your body does not shut down but instead goes through repair and maintenance of many important systems. Skimping on sleep can increase your risk of chronic disease and affect your immune and endocrine systems, which regulate hormones. In fact, a review article in the journal *Sleep Science* discussed how lack of sleep can negatively affect the hormones that control appetite and promote fat storage. Lack of sleep and being tired can also lead to overconsumption of food and a desire to eat unhealthy foods that include excess sugars and added fats.

Here are a few techniques for getting enough quality sleep:

- Step away from all screens at least 30 minutes before bedtime.

- Limit or eliminate screens in your bedroom. If your phone is also your alarm clock, set your phone so all other apps are limited during a set period each night.

- Have a consistent schedule for when you go to bed during the week.

- Incorporate regular exercise, which has been shown to improve sleep. Whenever possible, exercise earlier in the day or at least two hours before your scheduled bedtime.

- Set up your sleep environment to minimize noise, block out light, and create a cool environment. The National Sleep Foundation recommends a bedroom temperature of 60° to 67° Fahrenheit.

Reduce Stress

Everyone has stress in their life, and there is no way to eliminate it completely. The best approach is to try to reduce your stress and manage it. The hormones involved in the body's stress response were originally there to help with our fight-or-flight response, and those stress hormones encourage eating to fuel the need to either fight or flee.

In today's culture, our stress may not relate to fight or flight, but our hormones still respond that way because our bodies need to be ready at all times to deal with stressors. It is normal for the body to crave sugars and fats during stressful times, which can lead to weight gain.

While you have limited control over the cause of your stress, you can adjust how you respond to your stressors. Running late because you are stuck in traffic is a stressor, but what can you do about it? You can't get rid of the traffic, but you can change your reaction to it.

Try one or more of these techniques to deal with and reduce stress, even when you can't make large-scale changes:

- Adopt a mantra, such as "Will this matter in 30 days?" If the answer is no, let it go.

- Count to 10, or even 100, before responding or reacting to a stressful situation.

- Focus on breathing. Breathe in through your nose to the count of three and exhale to the count of three, visualizing stress leaving your body.

- Take a walk. Any form of exercise can help alleviate stress. Taking a walk around the block or the building is enough to remove yourself from a stressful situation and help calm both your body and your mind.

- Listen to music. Research published in the journal *PLOS One* suggests that music can have a beneficial effect on the human body and help with faster recovery from a stressful situation.

Feeling Ready

When preparing to make changes or implementing changes, an important factor of success is feeling ready. People tend to fear failure or aren't entirely sure what they need to do to make changes, so they often don't move forward. By reading this book, you are preparing yourself mentally for making the changes to achieve weight loss. You may already have taken some important steps, and reading this book is one of them.

If you have a slipup or setback, you are not a failure; you are simply finding out what isn't working and learning from it. You can make a different choice immediately, or at your very next meal.

You can be successful, and you can implement changes to lose weight. Say it out loud and believe it!

≡ EXERCISES IN THE PLAN ⟶

Everyone benefits from exercise, regardless of age or fitness level. Here's what you need to know about the different types of exercise.

Cardiovascular exercises, or "cardio," are activities that elevate your heart rate and strengthen your heart, which improve overall circulation. Strength training activities do strengthen your muscles, but they don't necessarily make them bigger. Flexibility, or stretching, can improve your balance and even reduce exercise-related injuries. The suggested exercises in this book are written for those just starting out. If you are regularly exercising already and looking for a change, you can increase the intensity of what is recommended here.

The recommended workouts are 30 minutes most days of the week, with a 60-minute workout on the weekend and one to two rest days. Rest days are just as important as the workout days because your body needs time to heal its muscles, nerves, and connective tissues.

Cardio workouts can include the following:

- Biking
- Dancing
- Following along with exercise videos
- Jogging
- Participating in group fitness classes

- Running
- Swimming
- Using machines such as the elliptical, treadmill, stationary bike, or stair stepper
- Walking

Strength workouts can include the following:

- Body weight exercises
- Exercising with dumbbells/hand weights
- Following along with exercise videos

- Using a medicine ball
- Using resistance bands
- Weight lifting

Flexibility/Stretching workouts can include the following:

- Pilates
- Following along with exercise videos

- Yoga

Loving Your Workouts

An important aspect of sticking with your workouts, besides finding something you enjoy, is to find ways to keep yourself motivated to do it regularly.

Setting up specific and achievable goals is key. Rather than just expressing the desire to exercise more or work out regularly, write down the specific number of days or minutes you will exercise each week. For example, set a goal of exercising for at least four days each week or doing at least 150 minutes of activity in the next seven days. Or sign up for a 5K run or fitness walk that is being held in 12 or more weeks. If it helps keep you motivated, consider giving yourself a reward, such as a pedicure or a massage, if you reach a certain goal.

Accountability partners and workout buddies can also inspire you to exercise more. An accountability partner may not be someone you exercise with, but if you share your workout goal with them, they can help hold you accountable. A workout buddy may be a person you exercise with, whether it is a friend or your partner, who agrees to go for a walk or attend a new fitness class with you. Joining a walking club or a running group provides an additional level of accountability and gives you ready-made workout buddies.

Music, podcasts, or audiobooks also can be invaluable tools in your workout plan, helping pump you up or just keep you entertained while you exercise. Finding ways to make exercise more enjoyable will make you more likely to do it and stick with it long term.

≡ WEEK 1: SHOPPING LIST ≡

The Week 1 Shopping List is extensive, but several items, especially the pantry items, will be used in subsequent weeks. Some items you will likely already have, so double-check what you need before heading out to the grocery store.

Pantry Items

- Artichoke hearts, not marinated—2 (14-ounce) jars or cans
- Baking powder—1 (8-ounce) container
- Basil, dried—1 container
- Beans, black, no-salt-added—1 (15 ¼-ounce) can
- Beans, Great Northern, no-salt-added—2 (15-ounce) cans
- Black pepper with grinder—1 jar
- Bread, whole-grain—1 (16-ounce) loaf
- Broth, 50 percent less sodium beef—2 (32-ounce) cartons

- Broth, reduced-sodium vegetable or chicken—2 (32-ounce) cartons
- Brown rice, precooked—1 (24-ounce) package
- Chili powder
- Cinnamon, ground
- Cooking spray, olive or canola oil—1 (8-ounce) can
- Corn, whole kernel—1 (8 ½-ounce) can
- Cumin, ground
- Dill, dried
- Enchilada sauce, red—2 (10-ounce) cans

- Garlic, jarred, minced—1 (8-ounce) jar (if not using fresh garlic)
- Garlic powder
- Lemon juice—1 (4½-ounce) container
- Maple syrup, pure—1 (12½-ounce) bottle
- Milk, evaporated, fat-free—1 (12-ounce) can
- Oats, old-fashioned—1 (42-ounce) package (will last the whole month)
- Oil, olive—1 (25½-ounce) container (will last the whole month)
- Oregano, dried
- Paprika, ground
- Salt
- Pasta, rotini, whole wheat—1 (16-ounce) package
- Peanut butter, natural—1 (16-ounce) container
- Pita chips, "naked" unsalted—1 (6¾-ounce) package

- Rosemary, dried
- Soy sauce, low-sodium (or tamari sauce)—1 (15-ounce) bottle
- Sugar, brown—1 (2-pound) package or smaller
- Thyme, dried
- Tomato paste, no-salt-added—1 (6-ounce) can
- Tomato sauce, no-salt-added—1 (15-ounce) can
- Tomatoes, whole, peeled, no-salt-added—1 (28-ounce) can
- Tortillas, corn—12 (6-inch)
- Trail mix—1 (26-ounce) package
- Tuna, albacore—1 (12-ounce) can
- Vanilla extract—1 (2-ounce) bottle
- Vinegar, rice wine—1 (12-ounce) bottle
- Water chestnuts, sliced—1 (8-ounce) can

Produce

- Apples (for snacks)—1 per snack, as desired
- Baby bok choy—1 pound
- Bananas (for snacks)—1 per snack, as desired
- Blueberries—2 cups
- Broccoli, florets—5 cups
- Carrots—1 pound
- Cauliflower—1 pound
- Celery—4 ounces

- Garlic—1 head
- Ginger—1 small "finger"
- Grapefruit—1 medium
- Lemon—2 medium
- Mushrooms, white or baby bella, sliced—4 ounces
- Onion, yellow—1¼ pounds
- Pepper, red bell—1 medium
- Potatoes, red small—½ pound
- Potatoes, russet—1½ pounds

- Raspberries—1 cup
- Snap peas—¼ pound
- Tomatoes, grape—12 ounces
- Tomatoes, large—2
- Zucchini—12 ounces

Meat and Fish

- Beef, ground, 95 percent lean—1 pound
- Beef, stew meat—1 pound
- Chicken, breasts, boneless, skinless—1 pound
- Chicken, thighs, boneless, skinless—1 pound
- Salmon, fillets—4 (6-ounce) fillets
- Turkey, breast, cooked, diced—¾ pound

Refrigerator Items

- Cheese, Cheddar, shredded— 1 (8-ounce package)
- Cheese, cottage, 2 percent fat— 1 (24-ounce) container
- Cheese, Monterey Jack, shredded— 1 (8-ounce) package
- Cheese, Parmesan, grated— 1 (6-ounce) package
- Cheese, string (for snacks)— 1 (12-ounce) package
- Cheese, Swiss, shredded— 1 (8-ounce) package
- Eggs, large—18 to 24
- Greek yogurt, plain, fat-free— 1 (32-ounce) container, plus additional for snacks
- Hummus—1 (10-ounce) container
- Milk, almond, dark chocolate—1½ gallons
- Milk, fat free—1½ gallons

Freezer Items

- Fruit, blueberries—1 (16-ounce) package (if fresh isn't available)
- Fruit, raspberries—1 (12-ounce) package (if fresh isn't available)
- Fruit, tart cherries— 1 (16-ounce) package
- Vegetables, butternut squash, diced—1 (10-ounce) package
- Vegetables, corn kernels— 1 (10-ounce) package (or canned)
- Vegetables, spinach, chopped— 1 (10-ounce) package
- Vegetables, sweet potatoes, diced— 1 (10-ounce) package

≡ WEEK 1: MEAL PLAN ≈

When referencing recipes in this book, the serving size is always one serving, as defined in each recipe. You'll find the cooking vessel used for each recipe in parentheses immediately following the recipe title.

WEEK 1	BREAKFAST	LUNCH	SNACK	DINNER	EXERCISE
DAY 1	Chocolate Cherry Smoothie (Blender)	Tuna Tomato Salad with White Beans (One Bowl)	½ grapefruit and 1 ounce string cheese	Cauliflower Potato Soup (Electric Pressure Cooker)	Cardio Machine Workout— 30 minutes
DAY 2	Sweet Potatoes with Sausage and Eggs (Skillet)	Leftover Cauliflower Potato Soup	¼ cup trail mix	Chicken and Rice with Broccoli and Squash (Casserole)	Resistance Training— 30-minute body weight workout
DAY 3	Chocolate Cherry Smoothie (Blender)	Leftover Chicken and Rice	6 ounces Greek yogurt	Cheeseburger Pasta Skillet	Rest Day or 30 minutes gentle stretching or yoga
DAY 4	Sweet Potatoes with Sausage and Eggs (Skillet)	Creamy Tomato Soup (Blender)	1 ounce (10 to 12) pita chips with 2 tablespoons hummus	Stacked Enchilada Casserole (Slow Cooker)	Cardio Outdoor Workout— 30 minutes
DAY 5	Chocolate Cherry Smoothie (Blender)	Leftover Enchilada Casserole	1 cup grape tomatoes and 1 cup snap peas	Salmon with Broccoli and Zucchini (Sheet Pan)	Resistance Training— 30-minute body weight workout
DAY 6	Mushroom Spinach Artichoke Breakfast Casserole (Slow Cooker)	Turkey and Vegetable Brown Rice Bowl (One Bowl)	1 apple and ¼ cup walnuts	Beef Stew (Soup Pot)	Cardio Workout— 60-minute walk or hike
DAY 7	Baked Oatmeal with Blueberries (Casserole)	1 slice whole-grain bread topped with 1 tablespoon peanut butter and 1 sliced banana	½ cup cottage cheese and 1 cup frozen raspberries	Lemon Chicken Thighs with Artichoke Hearts (Dutch Oven)	Rest Day

Before shopping this week, review this list for items you may have purchased last week, especially pantry items that come in larger quantities. Check your kitchen for these items to see if you should purchase more during your next shopping trip.

Pantry Items

- Beans, black, no-salt-added—1 (15¼-ounce) can
- Beans, kidney, no-salt-added—1 (15¼-ounce) can
- Beans, Great Northern, no-salt-added—1 (15½-ounce) can
- Bread, whole-grain English muffin—1 (6-count) package
- Broth, vegetable or chicken, low-sodium—1 (32-ounce carton)
- Juice, tomato or vegetable, low-sodium—24 ounces
- Herb/Spice, Old Bay or Cajun—1 container
- Honey—1 (12-ounce) jar
- Nuts, almonds—4 ounces
- Nuts, walnuts—4 ounces
- Oil, canola—1 (24-ounce) bottle
- Pasta, gnocchi—1 (12-ounce) package
- Salmon—1 (3-ounce) package
- Sauce, pizza—1 (24-ounce) jar
- Sunflower seeds—3 ounces
- Tomato paste, no-salt-added—1 (6-ounce) can

- Tomatoes, diced, no-salt-added—2 (14½-ounce) cans
- Tortilla chips—1 (1-ounce) bag
- Vinegar, balsamic—1 (8-ounce) bottle
- Vinegar, red wine—1 (12-ounce) bottle
- Worcestershire sauce—1 (10-ounce) bottle
- Basil, dried
- Black pepper
- Chili powder
- Cumin
- Garlic powder
- Maple syrup, pure
- Oats, old-fashioned
- Olive oil
- Oregano
- Pasta, rotini
- Peanut butter, natural
- Rosemary
- Salt
- Thyme
- Trail mix

Produce

- Apples, Granny Smith—2 medium
- Avocados—4
- Bananas—5
- Basil, fresh—1 bunch
- Beets—½ pound
- Blueberries—2 cups
- Carrots—½ pound
- Carrots, baby—½ pound
- Cilantro—1 bunch
- Cucumber—2
- Garlic—1 head
- Kale, chopped—1 pound
- Lemon—1 medium
- Mushrooms, white or baby bella, sliced—4 ounces
- Onion, red—1 small
- Onion, Vidalia—1 medium
- Onion, yellow—1 pound
- Pear—1
- Pepper, green bell—1 medium
- Pepper, jalapeño—1
- Pepper, red bell—4 medium
- Potatoes, sweet—2¼ pounds
- Spinach, baby—1 pound
- Tomatoes, grape—18 ounces
- Tomatoes, Roma—2
- Tomatoes, vine-ripened—2 pounds
- Zucchini or yellow squash—1 pound

Meat and Fish

- Beef, ground, 95 percent lean—1 pound
- Chicken, cooked, diced—6 pounds if buying whole rotisserie chicken or 2 pounds if buying the meat only, no bones
- Pork, tenderloin—1½ pounds
- Sausage, Cajun-style andouille—6 ounces
- Shrimp, large, frozen, shell on—1½ pounds
- Shrimp, medium, raw, peeled—1 pound
- Turkey, ground, lean—1 pound

Refrigerator Items

- Cheese, cheddar, shredded—½ cup
- Cheese, cottage, for snack—½ cup
- Cheese, Monterey Jack, shredded—½ cup
- Cheese, mozzarella, fresh—8 ounces
- Cheese, mozzarella, shredded—1 (8-ounce) package
- Eggs, large—10
- Greek yogurt, plain, fat-free—26 ounces, or 3¼ cups
- Greek yogurt for snacks
- Hummus
- Milk, fat-free—1¾ cups

Freezer Items

- Fruit, blueberries—2 cups
- Vegetables, corn on the cob—3- to 4-inch cob, 6 count
- Vegetables, mixed, including carrots, corn, green beans, and peas—1 (16-ounce) package

WEEK 2: MEAL PLAN

When referencing recipes in this book, the serving size is always one serving, as defined in each recipe. You'll find the cooking vessel used for each recipe in parentheses immediately following the recipe title.

WEEK 2	BREAKFAST	LUNCH	SNACK	DINNER	EXERCISE
DAY 8	Peanut Butter Banana Protein Bowl (One Bowl)	Gazpacho (Blender)	1 medium pear and 1 ounce cheddar cheese	Pork Tenderloin with Root Vegetables and Orange Honey Sauce (Sheet Pan)	Cardio Machine Workout— 30 minutes
DAY 9	Pan-Fried Oatmeal (Skillet)	Leftover Pork Tenderloin with Root Vegetables and Orange Honey Sauce	6 ounces Greek yogurt	Shrimp and Squash Skillet (Skillet)	Resistance Training— 30-minute body weight workout
DAY 10	Peanut Butter Banana Protein Bowl (One Bowl)	Chicken Caprese Bowl (One Bowl)	1 medium apple and ¼ cup walnuts	Sweet Potato Kale Soup (Dutch Oven)	Rest Day or 30 minutes gentle stretching or yoga
DAY 11	Pan-Fried Oatmeal (Skillet)	Leftover Sweet Potato Kale Soup	1 cup blueberries and ½ cup cottage cheese	Turkey Chili (Slow Cooker)	Cardio Outdoor Workout— 30 minutes
DAY 12	Peanut Butter Banana Protein Bowl (One Bowl)	Chunky Tortilla Soup (Blender)	¼ cup trail mix	Pizza Casserole (Dutch Oven)	Resistance Training— 30-minute body weight workout
DAY 13	Crustless Breakfast Quiche (Casserole)	3 ounces salmon (canned or pouch) with ½ cucumber and 2 ounces plain Greek yogurt	½ cup baby carrots and 2 tablespoons hummus	Chicken and Dumplings (Soup Pot)	Cardio Workout— 60-minute fitness class or video
DAY 14	Savory Oatmeal with Tomatoes and Avocados (Dutch Oven)	1 whole wheat English muffin topped with ½ avocado, mashed	¼ cup almonds	Shrimp Boil (Electric Pressure Cooker)	Rest Day

= WEEK 3: SHOPPING LIST =

Before shopping this week, review this list for items you may have purchased over the past two weeks, especially pantry items that come in larger quantities. Check your kitchen for these items to see if you should purchase more during your next shopping trip.

Pantry Items

- Almond butter—1 (12-ounce) jar
- Beans, black, no-salt-added—2 (15¼-ounce) cans
- Beans, Great Northern, no-salt-added—1 (15-ounce) can
- Beans, navy, no-salt-added—2 (15-ounce) cans
- Broth, vegetable or chicken, low-sodium—2 (32-ounce) cartons
- Chile, green, diced—1 (4-ounce) can
- Cornstarch—1 (6-ounce) container
- Garlic, jarred, minced—1 (8-ounce) jar
- Oil, sesame—1 (5-ounce) bottle
- Pineapple, chunks in its own juice—1 (20-ounce) can
- Quinoa, dry—1 (16-ounce) package
- Tomato paste, no-salt-added—1 (6-ounce) can
- Tomato sauce, no salt added—1 (15-ounce) can
- Tomatoes, crushed, no salt added—1 (28-ounce) can
- Tomatoes, diced, no salt added—2 (14½-ounce) cans

- Tomatoes, sun-dried—3 ounces
- Basil
- Black pepper
- Bread, whole grain
- Cumin
- Garlic powder
- Honey
- Maple syrup, pure
- Nuts, almonds
- Nuts, walnuts
- Oats, old-fashioned
- Oil, olive
- Oregano
- Paprika
- Peanut butter, natural
- Rosemary
- Soy sauce, low-sodium (or tamari sauce)
- Sugar, brown
- Trail mix
- Vinegar, rice wine

Produce

- Apples, green—6
- Asparagus—1 pound
- Broccoli, florets—1½ pounds
- Carrots—1¼ pounds
- Carrots, baby—½ pound
- Celery, diced—¾ pound
- Cucumber—2 medium
- Garlic—1 head
- Ginger, fresh—1 finger-size piece
- Kale, chopped—10 ounces
- Kiwi—3

- Nectarine—1 medium
- Onions—1 pound
- Pepper, green bell—1 medium
- Pepper, red bell—1 medium
- Pepper, yellow bell—1 medium
- Raspberries—½ pint
- Snap peas—½ pound
- Spinach, chopped—20 ounces
- Tomatoes, grape—½ pound
- Tomato, vine-ripened—1

Meat and Fish

- Beef, ground, 95 percent lean—1 pound
- Beef, tenderloin strips—1 pound
- Chicken, breast, boneless, skinless—3 pounds

- Roast beef, sliced—2 ounces
- Shrimp, cooked, peeled—1 pound
- Shrimp, medium, raw, peeled, tails removed—1 pound
- Turkey, sliced—2 ounces

Refrigerator Items

- Cheese, cottage—1 (16-ounce) tub
- Cheese, feta—1 (6-ounce) container
- Cheese, Mexican blend— 1 (8-ounce) package
- Cheese, string—1 package
- Eggs, large—14
- Greek yogurt—single-serving cup

- Milk, almond, plain—½ gallon
- Milk, fat-free—½ gallon
- Milk, soy, vanilla—½ gallon
- Pesto, premade—1 (6- to 8-ounce) container
- Tofu, extra-firm—16 ounces

Freezer Items

- Fruit, blueberries—2 cups

- Fruit, mixed berries—1 (16-ounce) package

WEEK 3: MEAL PLAN

When referencing recipes in this book, the serving size is always one serving, as defined in each recipe. You'll find the cooking vessel used for each recipe in parentheses immediately following the recipe title.

WEEK 3	BREAKFAST	LUNCH	SNACK	DINNER	EXERCISE
DAY 15	Apple Kiwi Spinach Smoothie (Blender)	Shrimp with Vegetables and Peanut Sauce (One Bowl)	½ cup cottage cheese and ½ cup berries	Chicken with Beans and Greens (Skillet)	Cardio Machine Workout—30 minutes
DAY 16	Quinoa Breakfast Bowls with Apples and Peanut Butter (Electric Pressure Cooker)	2 ounces sliced roast beef and 2 slices tomato on 1 slice whole-grain bread	¼ cup mixed nuts	Shrimp with Vegetables and Honey Soy Sauce (Dutch Oven)	Resistance Training—30-minute body weight workout
DAY 17	Apple Kiwi Spinach Smoothie (Blender)	Black Bean Soup (Blender)	6 ounces Greek yogurt	Beef with Broccoli (Slow Cooker)	Rest Day or 30 minutes gentle stretching or yoga
DAY 18	Tomato and Spinach Breakfast Stew (Soup Pot)	Leftover Beef with Broccoli	1 medium apple and 1 tablespoon almond butter	Tofu Curry (Skillet)	Cardio Outdoor Workout—30 minutes
DAY 19	Apple Kiwi Spinach Smoothie (Blender)	Pesto Quinoa Bowl (One Bowl)	1 nectarine and ¼ cup almonds	Lemon Chicken Orzo with Asparagus (Skillet)	Resistance Training—30-minute body weight workout
DAY 20	Blueberry Almond Oatmeal (Slow Cooker)	Leftover Lemon Chicken Orzo with Asparagus	¼ cup trail mix	Pasta e Fagioli (Soup Pot)	Cardio Workout—60-minute walk or hike outdoors
DAY 21	Spinach and Tomato Egg Breakfast (Electric Pressure Cooker)	2 ounces sliced turkey breast, 1 ounce string cheese, and 1 cup snap peas	½ cup baby carrots and ½ cup grape tomatoes	Sweet and Sour Chicken (Electric Pressure Cooker)	Rest Day

WEEK 4: SHOPPING LIST

Before shopping this week, review this list for items you may have purchased over the past three weeks, especially pantry items that come in larger quantities. Check your kitchen for these items to see if you should purchase more during your next shopping trip.

Pantry Items

- Beans, black, no-salt-added—1 (15¼-ounce) can
- Beans, chickpeas—2 (15½-ounce) cans
- Beans, Great Northern, no-salt-added—2 (15-ounce) cans
- Beets, sliced—2 (14½-ounce) cans
- Bread, cinnamon raisin bread—1 (16-ounce) loaf
- Bread, whole wheat pita—1 package
- Broth, vegetable or chicken, low-sodium—3 (32-ounce) cartons
- Chia seeds—2 ounces
- Corn, whole-kernel—1 (15¼-ounce) can
- Juice, grape—1 (12-ounce) bottle
- Juice, lemon
- Juice, lime
- Mustard, Dijon—1 (6- to 8-ounce) container
- Nuts, pecans—4 ounces
- Olives, kalamata—1 (9½-ounce) jar
- Pineapple, diced, in its own juice—1 (20-ounce) can
- Raisins—1 (12-ounce) package
- Tomato paste, no-salt-added—1 (6-ounce) can
- Tomato sauce, no-salt-added—1 (8-ounce) can
- Tomatoes, crushed, no-salt-added—1 (28-ounce) can
- Tomatoes diced, with green chilies—1 (10-ounce) can
- Tortillas, whole wheat—1 package
- Tuna—1 (3-ounce) pack
- Water chestnuts, sliced—1 (8-ounce) can
- Almond butter
- Basil, dried
- Black pepper
- Bread, whole grain
- Chili powder
- Cinnamon
- Coriander, 1 container
- Cumin
- Dill
- Garlic, jarred, minced
- Garlic powder
- Mixed nuts, unsalted
- Oats, old-fashioned
- Oil, olive
- Oregano

- Paprika
- Rosemary
- Sage, rubbed, 1 container
- Soy sauce, low-sodium (or tamari sauce)
- Tarragon

- Thyme
- Trail mix
- Turmeric, 1 container
- Vanilla extract
- Vinegar, balsamic
- Vinegar, red wine

Produce

- Apples, Granny Smith—4 medium
- Berries, mixed—3 cups
- Broccoli, florets—½ pound
- Carrots—¾ pound
- Celery sticks—4
- Cucumber—2 medium
- Garlic—1 head
- Green beans, fresh—12 ounces
- Kale, chopped—1 pound
- Mushrooms, white or baby bella, sliced—8 ounces

- Onion, red—3 medium
- Onion, white—¾ pound
- Onion, yellow—2 medium
- Pepper, green bell—1 medium
- Pepper, red bell—4 medium
- Potatoes, fingerling—½ pound
- Snow peas—½ cup
- Squash, butternut—1 pound
- Tomatoes, grape—1 pint
- Tomatoes, vine-ripened—2

Meat and Fish

- Beef, flank steak—1 pound
- Chicken, breasts, boneless, skinless—1½ pounds

- Pork, loin chops—1 pound
- Tilapia fillets—1½ pounds
- Turkey, breast tenderloins—1 pound

Refrigerator

- Cheese, cottage—1 (16-ounce) tub
- Cheese, feta—1 (6-ounce) container
- Cheese, Parmesan
- Cheese, queso fresco—1 (10-ounce) package

- Cheese, string—1 package
- Eggs—1 dozen
- Greek yogurt—single-serving cup
- Greek yogurt, plain fat-free—1 (32-ounce) container

WEEK 4: MEAL PLAN

When referencing recipes in this book, the serving size is always one serving, as defined in each recipe. You'll find the cooking vessel used for each recipe in parentheses immediately following the recipe title.

WEEK 4	BREAKFAST	LUNCH	SNACK	DINNER	EXERCISE
DAY 22	Overnight Oats (One Bowl)	White Bean and Corn Soup (Blender)	6 ounces Greek yogurt	Pork Loin with Apples and Onions (Dutch Oven)	Cardio Machine Workout— 30 minutes
DAY 23	Mixed Berry Soup (Soup Pot)	Leftover Pork Loin with Apples and Onions	¼ cup mixed nuts	Chicken Cacciatore (Slow Cooker)	Resistance Training— 30-minute body weight workout
DAY 24	Overnight Oats (One Bowl)	Mediterranean Salad (One Bowl)	1 medium apple and 1 ounce cheese	Baked Tilapia with Tomatoes and Green Beans (Sheet Pan)	Rest Day or 30 minutes gentle stretching or yoga
DAY 25	Mixed Berry Soup (Soup Pot)	Leftover Chicken Cacciatore	6 ounces Greek yogurt	Carrot Apple Soup with Turmeric (Soup Pot)	Cardio Outdoor Workout— 30 minutes
DAY 26	Overnight Oats (One Bowl)	Beet Soup (Blender)	4 celery sticks with 1 tablespoon nut butter	Turkey Stir-Fry (Skillet)	Resistance Training— 30-minute body weight workout
DAY 27	Black Bean and Egg "Burrito" Bowl (Dutch Oven)	3 ounces tuna with 2 teaspoons lemon juice on 1 slice whole-grain bread	¼ cup trail mix	Butternut Squash Chickpea Stew (Slow Cooker)	Cardio Workout— 60-minute group fitness class or video
DAY 28	French Toast Casserole (Electric Pressure Cooker)	Leftover Butternut Squash Chickpea Stew	1 cup diced pineapple and ¼ cup cottage cheese	Beef with Potatoes and Broccoli (Sheet Pan)	Rest Day

SETTING MEASURABLE GOALS

Set and track numerous goals that include more than just weight changes. Take measurements, including circumferences, at the start of the plan and at the end of the 28 days. Log your weight, energy, sleep, how you are feeling, and how your clothes fit each week. The changes may be small, but they are happening. Keeping a record of this will help keep you motivated.

Day/Date:

Weight:

Waist circumference:

Hip circumference:

Chest circumference:

Upper-arm circumference:

Thigh circumference:

Calf circumference:

On a scale of 1 to 10, how is my energy level?

On a scale of 1 to 10, how is my sleep?

On a scale of 1 to 10, how am I feeling overall?

Are my clothes fitting differently? If yes, how so?

Did I reach my exercise goal(s) for the week?

Notes about this week:

MEASURING YOUR RESULTS

Results and weight changes present in many ways. The number on the scale is one way to measure results, but don't forget to consider how you feel, how your clothes fit, how you are sleeping, and your overall energy level.

You can weigh yourself regularly, but try not to do so more than once a day since weight fluctuates throughout the day. If you want to weigh yourself daily, remember that results don't happen in one day but gradually instead. No matter how often you choose to weigh yourself, record your weight once a week, ideally on the same day and time each week. Weigh yourself first thing in the morning and choose a day midweek, such as a Wednesday or Thursday.

If you are doing this plan with your family, keep in mind that everybody is different and people lose weight at different rates. Some people will see differences immediately while others won't see changes until several weeks later. Avoid comparing yourself with others in your family; instead, focus on how your changes are happening and how you feel.

KEEP GOING!

It is completely normal for weight to fluctuate throughout the week and month. What may appear as a two-pound weight loss one day may be only a half-pound loss the next day. But don't get discouraged.

As long as you are persistent, you will see and feel results. This can be measured in pounds, but also in feelings: You may notice exercise is easier or that you're sleeping better. Long-term, sustainable weight loss takes time, so even if you do not see much weight loss after the first week, keep going. It will happen.

CELEBRATE NON-SCALE GAINS

Non-scale gains are the positive changes you're seeing or feeling that aren't related to the number on the scale. Even though the number on the scale is one indicator of success, your health is improving in many other ways. For example, many people don't realize that they can feel better than they do, but when they start eating less processed food and more whole foods, they do feel differently. Keeping exercise consistent will help you find muscles you never knew you had or perhaps forgot about.

Some other non-scale gains are noticing that a 30-minute walk is a lot easier than it used to be or that you're able to go farther without getting tired. Perhaps the distance you're walking is increasing. Make note of some of these things as you progress through your 28 days and beyond to serve as a reminder of how far you've come.

BEYOND THE PLAN

While this book features a 28-day plan, the idea is that this will continue past the 28 days to become part of your lifestyle that will continue for years. The 28-day plan gives you a jump start on eating healthier, making meals at home, and feeling better. Getting through the entire 28 days proves you can do it. By the end of the plan, you'll have the tools, you'll be used to this lifestyle, and your body will have adjusted to eating this way. To continue on this weight loss journey beyond the plan, keep monitoring your weight with a weekly check-in, balancing your macros, and maintaining a calorie deficit. When you reach your goal weight, maintain your calories to stay there. Don't skip exercise or overeat because you reached your goal.

Slow and steady weight loss takes time. Don't be discouraged if you don't lose weight every day or every week—it will happen at its own pace. Also, don't compare yourself to others. Pay attention to how *you* feel. The human body fluctuates naturally, so while some weeks may not result in much weight loss, other weeks may show better results. While water weight changes daily and can affect the number on the scale day-to-day, fat loss takes time and will show up on the scale over the course of weeks. Change takes time, so don't give up. You can do this, so keep going and be consistent.

Your Plan

You can continue to make your own plan after the 28 days outlined in this book. Continue to plan each week by creating your own combination of recipes from this book and perhaps even adding a new recipe each week using your favorite appliance or cooking vessel. Keep in mind that if you have a favorite breakfast or one-bowl salad or soup, it is okay to have the same recipe several days in a row.

When looking for or adding new recipes, check the nutrition information and look for options containing 300 to 400 calories per serving and about 20 grams of protein and complex carbohydrates that supply fiber from fruits, vegetables, and whole grains.

The more often you prepare and cook your meals at home, the more control you have over the overall calorie content you're consuming. You can also make sure you're getting the right balance of macros regularly.

Finally, don't let one day derail you from your overall goal or plan. If you slip up or if life events cause you to stray from your healthy routine, simply pick back up the following day.

Once you've completed the 28-day plan, use the template that follows to create your own ongoing plan.

WEEK OF:

DAY	BREAKFAST	LUNCH	SNACK	DINNER	EXERCISE
1					
2					
3					
4					
5					
6					
7					

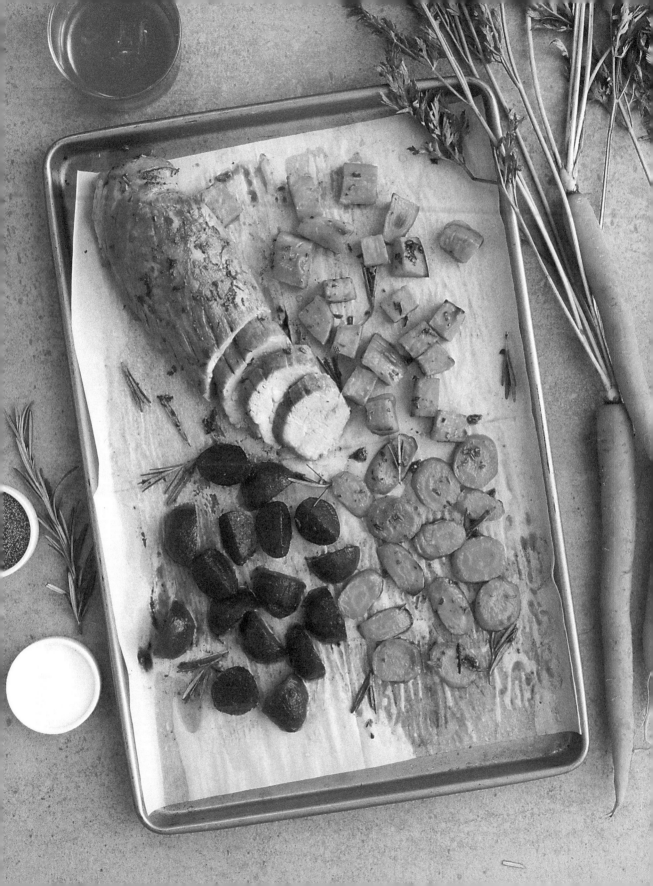

PART TWO

THE RECIPES

Pork Tenderloin with
Root Vegetables and
Orange Honey Sauce,
p. 148

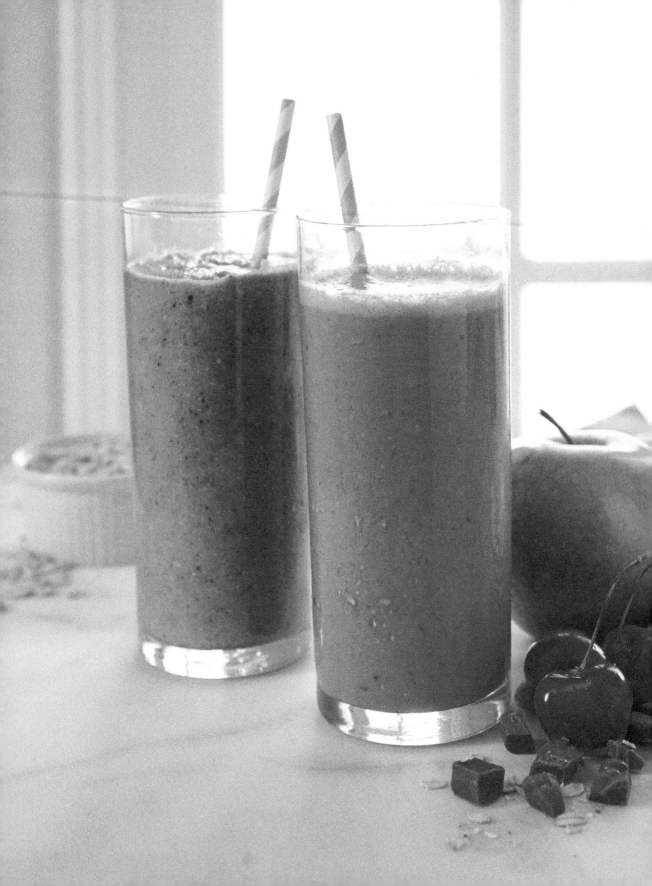

BLENDER

The recipes in this chapter are simple and easy, with no cooking required. Many are ready to consume directly from the blender, though some require refrigeration beforehand. You can find those additional steps in the directions.

Many of the soups may be prepared ahead of time and stored in the freezer for up to a few months. Depending on your schedule, you can make them over the weekend, store them in the refrigerator, and eat them throughout the week for quick grab-and-go meals.

As you make these recipes, keep in mind that blending speeds and times may vary based on your blender, so you can adjust them according to your personal preference.

**Apple Kiwi Spinach
Smoothie, p. 53**

BREAKFASTS

APPLE KIWI SPINACH SMOOTHIE 53

CHOCOLATE CHERRY SMOOTHIE 54

MAIN DISHES

BEET SOUP 55

BLACK BEAN SOUP 56

CHUNKY TORTILLA SOUP 57

CREAMY TOMATO SOUP 58

GAZPACHO 59

WHITE BEAN AND CORN SOUP 60

DESSERTS

AVOCADO CHOCOLATE PUDDING 61

STRAWBERRY CHEESECAKE 62

APPLE KIWI SPINACH SMOOTHIE

VEGETARIAN • VEGAN • GLUTEN-FREE • DAIRY-FREE • 30 MINUTES OR LESS

This delicious smoothie is packed with easy, healthy ingredients. The vitamin-rich spinach provides the smoothie's beautiful green color while the almond provides the protein and healthy fats you need for sustained energy. If you choose not to chop the spinach beforehand, pack the spinach leaves into the measuring cup and blend the smoothie for an additional 30 to 60 seconds. If you want a thicker smoothie, add a handful of ice to the blender or freeze the apple and kiwi the night before.

SERVES: 1

PREP TIME: 5 minutes

1 Granny Smith apple, core removed and sliced

1 kiwi, peeled

1 cup spinach leaves, chopped

1 cup vanilla soy milk

¼ cup almonds, unsalted

Put the apple, kiwi, spinach, milk, and almonds in a blender and blend for 30 to 90 seconds, or until well combined.

SUBSTITUTE! *You can use any type of nut, such as walnuts, for the almonds. And if you aren't a fan of the tart taste of green apples, you can choose a sweeter red one.*

Per serving: Calories: 423, Total Fat: 21g, Protein: 14g, Carbohydrates: 53g, Sugars: 35g, Fiber: 14g. Sodium: 216mg

CHOCOLATE CHERRY SMOOTHIE

VEGETARIAN • GLUTEN-FREE • 30 MINUTES OR LESS

Greek yogurt is higher in protein and lower in total carbohydrates than traditional yogurt. Adding plain Greek yogurt helps boost the protein content while also contributing probiotics and calcium. Using a flavored nut milk delivers a sweet taste while eliminating the need for unhealthy added sweeteners.

SERVES: *1*

PREP TIME: *5 minutes*

1 cup frozen tart cherries, pitted, unsweetened

1 cup dark chocolate almond milk

⅓ cup plain, fat-free Greek yogurt

¼ cup uncooked oats

Put the cherries, milk, yogurt, and oats in a blender and blend for 30 seconds, or until well combined. Serve immediately.

SUBSTITUTE! *Choose any fruit that you prefer. You can also choose fruit based on what's in season. Keep in mind that using frozen fruit makes a thicker smoothie, so when using fresh fruit, you can freeze overnight, if desired.*

Per serving: Calories: 332, Total Fat: 5g, Protein: 13g, Carbohydrates: 62g, Sugars: 44g, Fiber: 6g, Sodium: 228mg

BEET SOUP

VEGETARIAN · GLUTEN-FREE · NUT-FREE · DAIRY-FREE · 30 MINUTES OR LESS

Beets are packed with nutrients and low in calories. They also have a positive effect on blood pressure levels and contain other potential health benefits, including improving brain health and reducing the risk of cancer. This soup can be eaten cold, at room temperature, or warmed in a saucepan or microwave.

SERVES: *4*

PREP TIME: *10 minutes*

2 (14½-ounce) cans sliced beets

1 to 1½ cups low-sodium vegetable broth

½ cup chopped carrots

½ cup chopped onions

1 garlic clove, peeled, or 1 teaspoon jarred, minced garlic

1 teaspoon dried dill

½ teaspoon salt

¼ teaspoon freshly ground black pepper

Plain, fat-free Greek yogurt (optional)

1. Pour the liquid from the canned beets into a 4-cup liquid measuring cup. Add enough vegetable broth to the measuring cup to make 3 cups of liquid. Set aside.

2. Put the beets, carrots, onions, and garlic in a blender and pulse until a chunky consistency is reached.

3. Add the dill, salt, pepper, and 1 cup of the liquid to the blender. Cover and blend.

4. While blending, add the remaining 2 cups of liquid to the blender through the opening on the top of the lid. Blend until smooth.

5. Divide the soup into 4 bowls and top with yogurt (if using).

SUBSTITUTE! *For a heartier-tasting soup, substitute chicken broth for the vegetable broth.*

STORAGE: *Store in the refrigerator for up to four days or freeze individual servings for four to six months.*

Per serving: Calories: 110, Total Fat: 0g, Protein: 4g, Carbohydrates: 24g, Sugars: 18g, Fiber: 5g, Sodium: 512mg

BLACK BEAN SOUP

VEGETARIAN · GLUTEN-FREE · NUT-FREE · 30 MINUTES OR LESS

Beans have many health benefits: They are a good source of protein and fiber, and black beans, due to their dark color, are higher in antioxidants than other beans. Antioxidants help protect against cell damage and diseases associated with aging. This soup is also very versatile and may be served at room temperature or served warm. If serving warm, add the cheese after heating.

SERVES: *4*

PREP TIME: *10 minutes*

2 (15¼-ounce) cans black beans, no-salt-added, drained and rinsed

1 (14½-ounce) can diced tomatoes, no-salt-added

1 cup low-sodium vegetable broth

1 (4-ounce) can diced green chilies

1 teaspoon ground cumin

½ teaspoon salt

½ teaspoon garlic powder

½ cup shredded Mexican blend cheese, divided

1. Put the black beans, diced tomatoes with their juices, broth, green chiles, cumin, salt, and garlic powder in a blender.

2. Blend for 30 to 60 seconds, or until the desired consistency is reached.

3. Divide the soup into 4 bowls. Top each with 2 tablespoons of cheese.

SUBSTITUTE! *For a heartier-tasting soup, use chicken broth instead of vegetable broth.*

STORAGE: *Store in the refrigerator for up to 4 days or freeze individual servings for four to six months.*

Per serving: Calories: 260, Total Fat: 6g, Protein: 4g, Carbohydrates: 38g, Sugars: 4g, Fiber: 13g, Sodium: 529mg

CHUNKY TORTILLA SOUP

VEGETARIAN • GLUTEN-FREE • NUT-FREE • 30 MINUTES OR LESS

This blender soup calls for a jalapeño, a type of pepper that is high in capsaicin, which is associated with many health benefits. It works as an anti-inflammatory compound and may play a role in reducing obesity. If you are not used to "heat" or spice, use a smaller amount of jalapeño or skip it completely. This ingredient is one of the many used here that will aid in weight loss. This soup can be eaten cold, at room temperature, or warmed in a saucepan or microwave.

SERVES: *4*

PREP TIME: *10 minutes*

1 avocado, sliced

1 (15¼-ounce) can black beans, drained and rinsed

4 cilantro sprigs

1 red bell pepper, sliced

2 Roma tomatoes, quartered

1 jalapeño pepper stemmed and seeded

1 teaspoon garlic powder

½ teaspoon salt

1½ cups warm water, divided

½ cup shredded Monterey Jack cheese, divided

¼ cup plain, fat-free Greek yogurt, divided

¼ cup crushed unsalted or lightly salted tortilla chips, divided

1. Put the avocado, beans, cilantro, bell pepper, tomatoes, jalapeño, garlic powder, salt, and 1 cup of the warm water in a blender.

2. Blend on low speed for 15 to 30 seconds.

3. While blending, gradually add the remaining ½ cup of water through the opening on the top of the lid.

4. Increase the speed and continue blending in 30-second increments until the soup is well combined and has a chunky texture (or to your desired consistency). Add more or less water as desired.

5. Divide the soup into 4 bowls or mugs. Top each with 2 tablespoons of cheese, 1 tablespoon of yogurt, and 1 tablespoon of crushed tortilla chips.

SUBSTITUTE! *If you're out of black beans or just looking to increase your potassium intake, one (15¼-ounce) can of pinto beans may be used instead.*

STORAGE: *Store individual servings in the refrigerator for up to four days or in the freezer for four to six months. Add the cheese, yogurt, and tortilla chips before serving.*

Per serving: Calories: 264, Total Fat: 13g, Protein: 12g, Carbohydrates: 28g, Sugars: 10g, Fiber: 3g, Sodium: 403mg

CREAMY TOMATO SOUP

VEGETARIAN · GLUTEN-FREE · NUT-FREE · 30 MINUTES OR LESS

This tomato soup is rich in lycopene, a substance found in tomatoes that is connected with reduced risk of cancer and heart disease. It is best absorbed by the body when heated and combined with a little bit of healthy fat. Accordingly, using canned tomatoes, which have already been heated, and olive oil boost the lycopene's ability to fight disease.

SERVES: *4*

PREP TIME: *10 minutes*

1 (28-ounce) can whole, peeled tomatoes

1 (6-ounce) can tomato paste

¼ cup olive oil

2 garlic cloves, peeled, or 2 teaspoons jarred, minced garlic

1 teaspoon dried oregano

1 teaspoon dried basil

1 (12-ounce) can fat-free evaporated milk

¼ cup grated Parmesan cheese, divided

1. Put the canned tomatoes with their juice, tomato paste, olive oil, garlic, oregano, and basil in a blender.

2. Blend on low speed for 10 to 20 seconds, then increase to medium speed.

3. While blending, add the evaporated milk through the opening on the top of the lid.

4. Divide the soup into 4 bowls or mugs. Top each with 1 tablespoon of cheese.

SUBSTITUTE! *Unflavored nut or soy milk may be substituted for the milk for a vegan or nondairy option.*

STORAGE: *Store in the refrigerator for up to four days. If you're using broth in place of the milk, freeze for four to six months. Don't freeze the soup if it contains milk.*

Per serving: Calories: 320, Total Fat: 21g, Protein: 12g, Carbohydrates: 25g, Sugars: 18g, Fiber: 4g, Sodium: 479mg

GAZPACHO

GLUTEN-FREE · NUT-FREE · DAIRY-FREE

Gazpacho is a tomato-based soup containing a mix of vegetables, blended and served cold. A classic of southern Spain, it can be a main dish or divided into smaller servings as a starter or side with grilled fish or chicken.

SERVES: *4*

PREP TIME: *15 minutes*

TOTAL TIME: *4 hours, 15 minutes*

2 pounds vine-ripened tomatoes, quartered

1 cucumber, peeled and seeded

1 green bell pepper, quartered

1 small red onion, quartered

2 garlic cloves, peeled, or 2 teaspoons jarred, minced garlic

2 tablespoons olive oil

2 tablespoons red wine vinegar

1 tablespoon Worcestershire sauce

½ teaspoon freshly ground black pepper

1. Put the tomatoes, cucumber, green pepper, onion, and garlic in a blender.

2. Blend on low speed. When it begins to liquefy, increase to medium speed.

3. While blending, add the olive oil, red wine vinegar, Worcestershire sauce, and black pepper through the opening on the top of the lid. Continue to blend the ingredients for about 30 seconds.

4. Divide the soup into 4 bowls or mugs and chill for 4 hours.

STORAGE: *Store in the refrigerator for up to four days or freeze individual servings for four to six months.*

Per serving: Calories: 137, Total Fat: 8g, Protein: 3g, Carbohydrates: 17g, Sugars: 10g, Fiber: 4g, Sodium: 56mg

WHITE BEAN AND CORN SOUP

VEGETARIAN • VEGAN • GLUTEN-FREE • NUT-FREE • DAIRY-FREE • 30 MINUTES OR LESS

Corn is a whole grain that is rich in vitamin C, fiber, and plant chemicals that support eye health. Combined with the white beans and bell pepper, this soup is loaded with filling fiber. Depending on your preference, it can be eaten cold, at room temperature, or warmed in a saucepan or microwave.

SERVES: *4*

PREP TIME: *10 minutes*

2 (15½-ounce) cans white beans, drained and rinsed

1 (15¼-ounce) can whole-kernel corn

1 red bell pepper, sliced

1 cup vegetable broth

2 teaspoons lime juice

1 teaspoon dried thyme

1 teaspoon garlic powder

½ teaspoon salt

¼ teaspoon freshly ground black pepper

1. Put the white beans, corn with its juice, bell pepper, and vegetable broth in a blender and blend for 20 seconds.

2. Add the lime juice, thyme, garlic powder, salt, and pepper, and blend for 10 to 20 seconds.

3. Divide the soup into 4 bowls and serve.

SUBSTITUTE! *For a heartier-tasting soup, substitute chicken broth for the vegetable both.*

STORAGE: *Store in the refrigerator for up to four days or in the freezer for four to six months.*

Per serving: Calories: 246, Total Fat: 2g, Protein: 14g, Carbohydrates: 45g, Sugars: 6g, Fiber: 17g, Sodium: 811mg

AVOCADO CHOCOLATE PUDDING

VEGETARIAN · VEGAN · GLUTEN-FREE · NUT-FREE · DAIRY-FREE · 30-MINUTES OR LESS

This rich chocolate pudding is a healthier alternative to traditional chocolate mousse made with heavy cream. Swapping avocado for the cream gives it a better fat profile and contains more nutrients, such as fiber, vitamin E, and potassium.

SERVES: 6

....

PREP TIME: *5 minutes*

....

TOTAL TIME: *1 hour, 5 minutes*

....

2 whole avocados

1 cup unsweetened cocoa powder

½ cup pure maple syrup

½ cup coconut milk

1. Peel and dice the avocados and put them in a blender.

2. Add the cocoa power, maple syrup, and coconut milk. Blend until smooth, stopping to scrape the sides as needed to incorporate all of the cocoa.

3. Divide the mousse into 6 bowls and chill for 1 hour, or until firm.

SUBSTITUTE! *Depending on what you have on hand, vanilla-flavored almond or soy milk may be used in place of the coconut milk. Using flavored milk, such as vanilla, adds more flavor without having to use additional maple syrup.*

STORAGE: *Store covered in the refrigerator for up to three days.*

Per serving: Calories: 244, Total Fat: 16g, Protein: 4g, Carbohydrates: 32g, Sugars: 17g, Fiber: 9g, Sodium: 13mg

STRAWBERRY CHEESECAKE

VEGETARIAN • NUT-FREE • 30 MINUTES OR LESS

This decadent cheesecake is made with Neufchâtel cheese, which is virtually the same as cream cheese except that it is lower in calories and total fat and higher in protein. Unless someone is doing a side-by-side comparison with cream cheese, most people will not know that one was used instead of the other. You can find Neufchâtel cheese next to cream cheese in the grocery store. Give it a try and wow your family with this healthy take on a classic favorite dessert.

SERVES: *6*

PREP TIME: *10 minutes*

TOTAL TIME: *1 hour, 10 minutes*

1 (8-ounce) package
   Neufchâtel
   cheese, softened

1 cup part-skim
   ricotta cheese

½ cup pure maple syrup

1 teaspoon vanilla extract

3 sheets graham crackers
   or ⅓ cup graham
   cracker crumbs

1½ cups sliced fresh
   strawberries, divided

1. Put the Neufchâtel cheese and ricotta in a blender.

2. Blend on low speed for 30 to 60 seconds, then increase to medium speed.

3. While blending, add the maple syrup and vanilla through the opening on the top of the lid. Stop the blender and scrape the sides as needed to ensure that all ingredients are incorporated.

4. Put the graham crackers in a zip-top bag and crush into crumbs with your hands or a rolling pin.

5. Put 1 tablespoon of graham cracker crumbs into each of 6 glasses or small bowls.

6. Pour about ⅓ cup of the cheese mixture over the graham cracker crumbs in each container.

7. Chill in the refrigerator for at least 1 hour.

8. Top each dessert with ¼ cup of sliced strawberries.

SUBSTITUTE! *It isn't always easy to find fresh strawberries, so you can use frozen strawberries or other fresh seasonal berries instead.*

STORAGE: *If you keep this dessert past the 1-hour chilling time, cover with plastic wrap until you're ready to serve.*

Per serving: Calories: 307, Total Fat: 14g, Protein: 10g, Carbohydrates: 37g, Sugars: 22g, Fiber: 2g, Sodium: 345mg

CHAPTER 3: NOTES

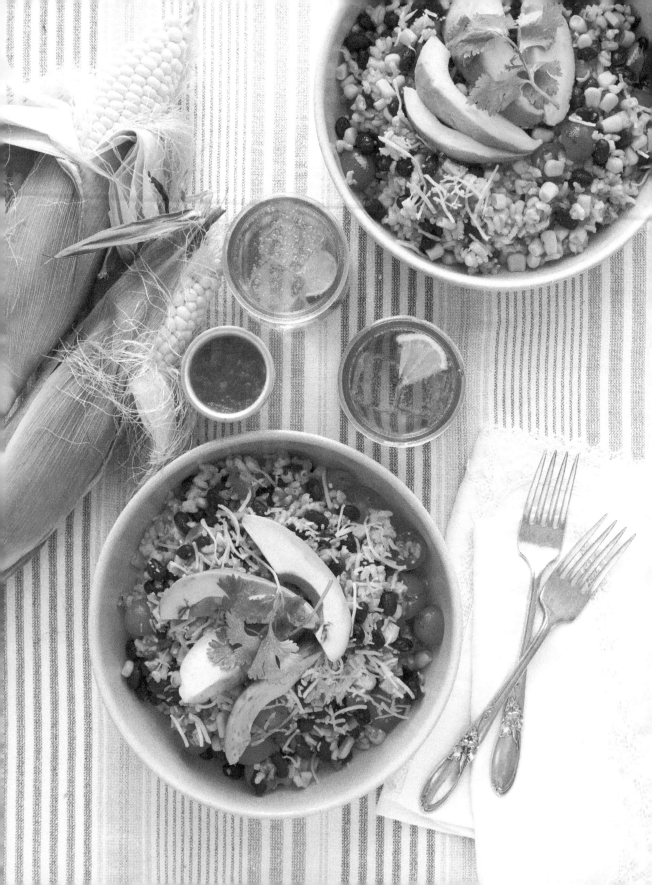

ONE BOWL

While the vessel used in this chapter is referred to as a "bowl," you'll find recipes that use a cereal bowl, a large salad bowl, or even a mason jar. Because the main vessel is a bowl, most of the recipes in this chapter are uncooked, though a microwave is required in some cases. For those recipes, make sure that the bowl or container is microwave-safe.

Because the recipes do not require cooking, they often include common canned or prepared meats, such as canned tuna or rotisserie chicken, along with canned beans and precooked grains. You can find precooked grains such as brown rice and quinoa in the same aisle as uncooked grains or in the freezer section of your grocery store.

Veggie Burrito
Bowl, p. 71

BREAKFASTS

OVERNIGHT OATS 67

PEANUT BUTTER BANANA PROTEIN BOWL 68

MAIN DISHES

MEDITERRANEAN SALAD 69

PESTO QUINOA BOWL 70

VEGGIE BURRITO BOWL 71

SHRIMP WITH VEGETABLES AND
PEANUT SAUCE 72

TUNA TOMATO SALAD WITH
WHITE BEANS 73

CHICKEN CAPRESE BOWL 74

TURKEY AND VEGETABLE BROWN
RICE BOWL 75

DESSERTS

KEY LIME PIE FROZEN YOGURT 76

OVERNIGHT OATS

VEGETARIAN · VEGAN · GLUTEN-FREE · DAIRY-FREE · 30 MINUTES OR LESS

Keep the combined dry ingredients on hand and just add the liquid the night before. You can make multiple individual servings in reusable containers with lids or mason jars. Overnight Oats can be eaten chilled or warm—just microwave for about two minutes.

SERVES: *1*

PREP TIME: *5 minutes*

COOK TIME: *2 minutes, plus*
chilling overnight

½ cup old-fashioned
 rolled oats

2 tablespoons raisins

2 tablespoons
 chopped pecans

1 tablespoon chia
 seeds (optional)

1 cup vanilla soy milk

1. Put the oats, raisins, pecans, and chia seeds (if using) in a mason jar or small container with a lid.

2. Add the soy milk.

3. Cover and put in the refrigerator overnight.

4. Serve cold in the container or heat in the microwave, uncovered, for 2 minutes, if desired. Stir before eating.

SUBSTITUTE! *To add a bit more flavor and sweetness, use 2 tablespoons of dried fruit or ½ cup of fresh fruit in place of the raisins. You can also use 2 tablespoons of another nut instead of the pecans for a slightly different flavor profile.*

STORAGE: *For optimal freshness, eat within one day of adding milk or fresh fruit.*

SHORTCUT! *To save some time, you can make the oats in individual containers without the milk and store them in the pantry. Simply add the milk and move the container to the refrigerator the night before eating.*

Per serving: Calories: 370, Total Fat: 15g, Protein: 11g, Carbohydrates: 53g, Sugars: 19g, Fiber: 6g, Sodium: 124mg

PEANUT BUTTER BANANA PROTEIN BOWL

VEGETARIAN · GLUTEN-FREE · 30 MINUTES OR LESS

This breakfast bowl contains 20 grams of protein, which will help sustain you throughout the morning. If you exercise in the morning, split this bowl into two servings and have half before your workout for fuel and the other half after your workout for your recovery.

SERVES: 1

PREP TIME: 5 minutes

1 tablespoon natural peanut butter

¾ cup (6 ounces) plain, fat-free Greek yogurt

1 medium banana, sliced

1. In a small glass or ceramic cereal bowl, melt the peanut butter in the microwave on medium power for 20 to 30 seconds.

2. Add the yogurt and stir until well combined and smooth.

3. Add the sliced banana and mix to incorporate.

SUBSTITUTE! *With 1 tablespoon of almond butter you get twice the fiber and more grams per serving of heart-healthy monounsaturated fat than from peanut butter.*

SHORTCUT! *To save some time, mix several servings of the peanut butter and yogurt and store in individual containers for up to one week. When you're ready to eat the protein bowl, simply grab a container and top with the sliced banana for a quick and easy breakfast.*

Per serving: Calories: 306, Total Fat: 8g, Protein: 23g, Carbohydrates: 38g, Sugars: 21g, Fiber: 4g, Sodium: 4mg

MEDITERRANEAN SALAD

VEGETARIAN • NUT-FREE • 30 MINUTES OR LESS

This colorful salad combines flavors from the countries of the Mediterranean. The Mediterranean diet is considered one of the healthiest diets in the world, with a variety of fruits, vegetables, whole grains, and legumes along with moderate amounts of olive oil and lean protein. There are variations depending on the country, and this recipe uses many of their best flavors.

SERVES: *4*

PREP TIME: *15 minutes*

¼ cup red wine vinegar

2 tablespoons olive oil

1 tablespoon fresh oregano or 1 teaspoon dried oregano

1 teaspoon lemon juice

½ teaspoon salt

¼ teaspoon pepper

1 (15½-ounce) can chickpeas, drained and rinsed

2 medium cucumbers, sliced

2 vine-ripened tomatoes, chopped

¼ cup kalamata olives, chopped

½ cup (2 ounces) feta cheese, crumbled

4 whole wheat pita pockets (optional)

1. In a large bowl, combine the red wine vinegar, olive oil, oregano, lemon juice, salt, and pepper. Whisk to combine.

2. Add the chickpeas, cucumbers, tomatoes, olives, and feta cheese. Toss to combine.

3. Divide into individual bowls or fill each of the pita pockets (if using) for a handheld meal.

SUBSTITUTE! *Depending on what you have on hand, you can use 1 cup halved grape or cherry tomatoes instead of chopped tomatoes.*

STORAGE: *You can keep leftovers in the refrigerator for up to three days. Make sure to toss the salad again before serving.*

Per serving: Calories: 333, Total Fat: 15g, Protein: 12g, Carbohydrates: 42g, Sugars: 8g, Fiber: 9g, Sodium: 733mg

PESTO QUINOA BOWL

VEGETARIAN • GLUTEN-FREE • 30 MINUTES OR LESS

Pesto, a sauce traditionally made with basil, salt, garlic, olive oil, pine nuts, and Parmesan cheese, is the standout flavor of this dish. Herbs, garlic, nuts, and olive oil each have tremendous health benefits, so combining them here provides a big boost of nutrients. This recipe uses premade pesto to cut down on prep time. Pesto is readily available and easy to find in jars in the pasta sauce aisle or the refrigerated section in your grocery store.

SERVES: 4

PREP TIME: 10 minutes

8 ounces precooked quinoa

⅓ cup pesto

3 ounces sun-dried
  tomatoes, chopped

6 ounces fresh
  spinach, chopped

¼ cup chopped walnuts

1. Reheat the quinoa according to package directions.

2. In a medium bowl, combine the pesto sauce, sun-dried tomatoes, and fresh spinach.

3. Add the reheated quinoa to the bowl, tossing to mix well.

4. Top with the walnuts, divide into 4 bowls, and serve.

SUBSTITUTE! *While walnuts are a healthier option, you can use pine nuts instead for a slightly different flavor.*

STORAGE: *Store any leftovers in the refrigerator for up to three days. Toss again before serving.*

Per serving: Calories: 266, Total Fat: 15g, Protein: 10g, Carbohydrates: 27g, Sugars: 10g, Fiber: 6g, Sodium: 604mg

VEGGIE BURRITO BOWL

VEGETARIAN · GLUTEN-FREE · NUT-FREE · 30 MINUTES OR LESS

This burrito bowl is a twist on a classic Mexican favorite. It's full of satisfying brown rice, antioxidant-rich black beans, and cilantro. People either love or hate fresh cilantro, so if you love it, add more, and if you don't, skip it. It won't affect the nutrition.

SERVES: *4*

PREP TIME: *10 minutes*

1 (8-ounce) package precooked brown rice

3 tablespoons fresh cilantro

1 tablespoon lime juice

1 (15½-ounce) can black beans, drained and rinsed

1 (15-ounce) can whole-kernel corn, drained

2 cups halved grape or cherry tomatoes

¾ cup salsa

½ cup shredded Mexican blend cheese, divided

2 avocados, sliced

1. In a large bowl, combine the brown rice, cilantro, and lime juice.

2. Add the black beans, corn, and tomatoes. Top with the salsa and mix.

3. Divide into four small bowls. Top each serving with 2 tablespoons of cheese and one-quarter of the avocado slices.

SUBSTITUTE! *If you don't have time to run to the store, you can easily turn to your pantry to adapt this recipe. Simply use one (15½-ounce) can of pinto beans or 2 cups of rotisserie chicken in place of the black beans.*

STORAGE: *Store the salad for up to four days in the refrigerator, adding the avocado right before serving.*

SHORTCUT! *Make this dish on prep day (adding the avocado right before serving) and have this salad for lunch during the week.*

Per serving: Calories: 405, Total Fat: 20g, Protein: 15g, Carbohydrates: 49g, Sugars: 8g, Fiber: 16g, Sodium: 408mg

SHRIMP WITH VEGETABLES AND PEANUT SAUCE

DAIRY-FREE • 30 MINUTES OR LESS

Protein-packed peanut sauce can be used on many savory dishes, but it's especially delicious with shrimp, chicken, and vegetables. It's also a great dressing or dipping sauce. While most peanut sauces come with a little kick, you can easily adjust the red pepper flakes in this to the level of spice you prefer.

SERVES: *4*

PREP TIME: *15 minutes*

⅓ cup creamy peanut butter

3 tablespoons low-sodium soy sauce

1 tablespoon lime juice

1 tablespoon pure maple syrup

1 teaspoon red pepper flakes

2 tablespoons water

1 pound cooked shrimp, peeled and tails removed

2 cups broccoli florets

2 cucumbers, chopped

1 cup shredded carrots

1 yellow bell pepper, diced

1. In a large ceramic or glass bowl, heat the peanut butter in the microwave on medium for 30 seconds.
2. Add the soy sauce, lime juice, maple syrup, and red pepper flakes. Whisk until it forms a thin sauce. Add up to 2 tablespoons of water to thin the sauce so it will coat the shrimp and vegetables.
3. Add the shrimp, broccoli, cucumbers, carrots, and bell pepper. Toss to distribute the peanut sauce evenly.
4. Divide into 4 small bowls and serve.

SUBSTITUTE! *If you're looking for a gluten-free option, you can use tamari sauce instead of soy sauce.*

STORAGE: *This dish can be stored in the refrigerator for up to three days. Peanut sauce will become thicker when refrigerated but will thin out once reheated.*

SHORTCUT! *To save some time, you can purchase precooked shrimp in the prepared foods section of your grocery store. You can also make this recipe on prep day and serve it through-out the week for a quick and easy dinner your whole family will love.*

Per serving: Calories: 341, Total Fat: 13g, Protein: 35g, Carbohydrates: 25g, Sugars: 12g, Fiber: 5g, Sodium: 1,074mg

TUNA TOMATO SALAD WITH WHITE BEANS

GLUTEN-FREE • NUT-FREE • DAIRY-FREE • 30 MINUTES OR LESS

Tuna, the featured ingredient in this dish, is a good source of protein and healthy omega-3 fats. To get these healthy fats, make sure you're purchasing albacore tuna and not chunk light tuna. While albacore tuna is sold in cans like chunk light tuna, it is a lighter-colored fish with a firmer texture and milder flavor. When shopping, remember that the healthy fat is in the fish, not the oil the fish is sometimes packed in, so choose tuna packed in water.

SERVES: 4

PREP TIME: *15 minutes*

3 tablespoons lemon juice

¼ cup olive oil

1 teaspoon dried rosemary or 1 tablespoon chopped fresh rosemary

1 teaspoon salt

½ tablespoon freshly ground black pepper

2 (15-ounce) cans white beans, drained and rinsed

1 (12-ounce) can albacore tuna in water, drained

2 large tomatoes, chopped

1. In a large bowl, whisk together the lemon juice, olive oil, rosemary, salt, and pepper.

2. Add the white beans, tuna, and tomatoes, breaking up the tuna with a fork. Toss to combine.

3. Divide into 4 bowls and serve.

SUBSTITUTE! *Depending on what you have on hand, you can use 1½ cups of halved grape or cherry tomatoes in place of chopped tomatoes.*

STORAGE: *Store in the refrigerator until you're ready to serve. Note that this dish may be stored for up to three days. Remember to toss again before serving.*

Per serving: Calories: 451, Total Fat: 15g, Protein: 35g, Carbohydrates: 46g, Sugars: 3g, Fiber: 18g, Sodium: 631mg

CHICKEN CAPRESE BOWL

GLUTEN-FREE • NUT-FREE • 30 MINUTES OR LESS

Caprese salad is a three-ingredient wonder salad from Italy: fresh tomatoes, mozzarella, and basil, and it's red, white, and green like the Italian flag. This bowl features chicken to make it a more filling main dish that tastes just as good the next day as leftovers. The bonus is this versatile dish can easily be served in smaller portions as an appetizer or starter.

SERVES: *4*

PREP TIME: *15 minutes*

3 tablespoons olive oil

3 tablespoons
  balsamic vinegar

1 teaspoon salt

½ teaspoon freshly ground
  black pepper

2 cups diced rotisserie
  chicken breast

4 vine-ripened tomatoes,
  coarsely chopped

8 ounces fresh mozzarella,
  cut into bite-size pieces

1 bunch fresh basil

1. In a large bowl, whisk together the olive oil, balsamic vinegar, salt, and pepper.

2. Add the diced chicken, tomatoes, and mozzarella.

3. Choose 8 to 10 large basil leaves and rip them by hand, then add to the bowl.

4. Toss the ingredients until mixed and serve immediately.

SUBSTITUTE! *For a vegetarian alternative, use one 15¼-ounce can of white beans or chickpeas, drained and rinsed, in place of the chicken.*

STORAGE: *Store in the refrigerator for up to three days. To better incorporate the flavors, toss again before serving.*

Per serving: Calories: 400, Total Fat: 26g, Protein: 35g, Carbohydrates: 5g, Sugars: 3g, Fiber: 1g, Sodium: 821mg

TURKEY AND VEGETABLE BROWN RICE BOWL

NUT-FREE • DAIRY-FREE • 30 MINUTES OR LESS

Bok choy is the vegetable known as Chinese cabbage. It is found in the produce section of most grocery stores. It can be eaten raw or cooked, and baby bok choy has a mild flavor. Bok choy is a good source of vitamin A, vitamin C, and vitamin K, with very few calories. Other Asian flavors such as soy sauce, rice wine vinegar, ginger, and water chestnuts round out this dish.

SERVES: *4*

PREP TIME: *15 minutes*

3 tablespoons soy sauce

1 tablespoon rice wine vinegar

1 tablespoon brown sugar

1 teaspoon freshly grated ginger or ¼ teaspoon dried ginger

1 (8-ounce) package precooked brown rice

1 pound baby bok choy, chopped

3 cups (12 ounces) precooked turkey breast, diced

1 (8-ounce) can sliced water chestnuts, drained

1 cup shredded carrots

1. In a large bowl, whisk together the soy sauce, rice wine vinegar, brown sugar, and ginger.

2. Add the brown rice, bok choy, turkey, water chestnuts, and shredded carrots.

3. Toss together to mix and distribute the dressing.

4. Divide into 4 bowls and serve.

SUBSTITUTE! *If your grocery store doesn't carry precooked turkey, you can substitute rotisserie chicken breast for the turkey.*

STORAGE: *Store in the refrigerator for up to two days.*

Per serving: Calories: 303, Total Fat: 2g, Protein: 30g, Carbohydrates: 41g, Sugars: 5g, Fiber: 2g, Sodium: 621mg

KEY LIME PIE FROZEN YOGURT

VEGETARIAN • NUT-FREE • 30 MINUTES OR LESS

Is there anything quite as satisfying as a delicious, tart Key lime pie? How about the fact that Key limes have been shown to help fight diabetes, aging, and more? This healthy twist on a classic dessert created in (and named for) the Florida Keys will leave you feeling both satisfied and confident in your dietary decisions. If you don't have access to Key limes or Key lime juice in your local grocery store, try lime juice. Fresh lime juice has a more intense flavor, but bottled lime juice will do just fine and saves time.

SERVES: *4*

PREP TIME: *10 minutes*

TOTAL TIME: *2 hours, 10 minutes*

2 sheets graham crackers or ¼ cup graham cracker crumbs

16-ounces vanilla fat-free Greek yogurt

⅓ cup Key lime juice, divided

1. Put the graham crackers in a zip-top bag and crush with your hands or a rolling pin. Set aside.

2. Put the yogurt in a medium glass or stainless steel bowl.

3. Add approximately half of the lime juice to the yogurt and mix well. Add the remaining lime juice and mix until fully blended.

4. Add the crushed graham crackers to the yogurt mixture and stir until evenly incorporated.

5. Divide into 4 bowls and freeze for at least 2 hours.

6. Allow the yogurt to sit outside the freezer for 5 to 10 minutes before serving.

STORAGE: *This may be stored in individual serving containers or in a single container. If stored in a single container, it will take longer to freeze through. Also, because this is a fat-free yogurt with added juice, it may freeze more solid than traditional ice creams or frozen yogurt. This dish can be stored in the freezer for up to two months.*

Per serving: Calories: 174, Total Fat: 2g, Protein: 10g, Carbohydrates: 30g, Sugars: 17g, Fiber: 1g, Sodium: 176mg

CHAPTER 4: NOTES

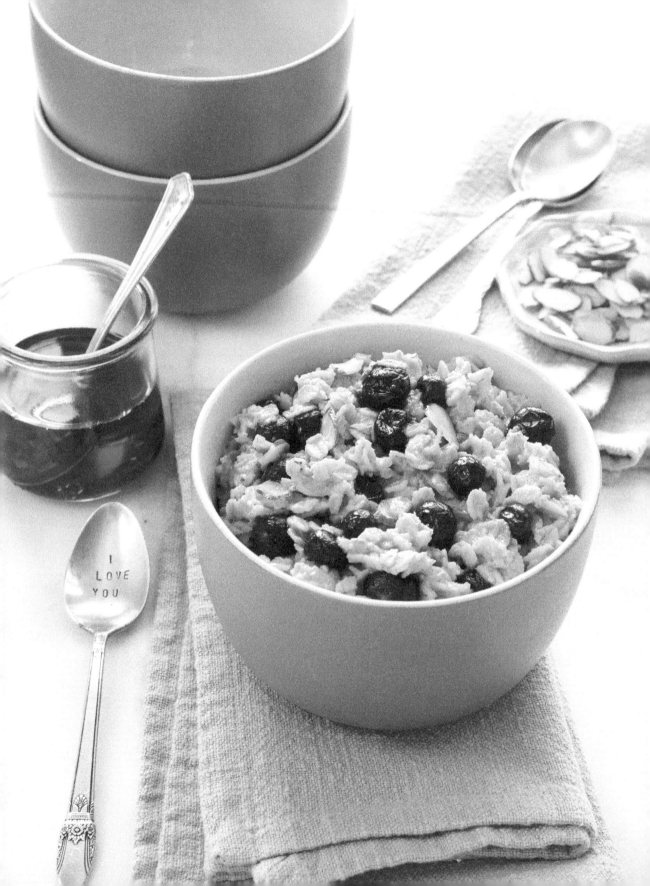

CHAPTER 5

SLOW COOKER

When making these recipes in the slow cooker, most ingredients will go directly into the pot in the order they are listed. All you'll need to do is set the timer and walk away for several hours until it's time to eat. In some cases, a final ingredient or two is added at the end to avoid over-cooking, so be sure to read the recipes all the way through.

If your slow cooker does not have a sauté or browning feature that some of the recipes call for, this step can be skipped. Sautéing or browning food first helps bring out a different flavor, but it is not essential.

Ideally, a slow cooker will have both "delay start" and "warm" functions so that ingredients can be assembled in the slow cooker and set to start midday for the allotted time. The warm function keeps the food warm without continuing to cook, so you don't have to serve immediately when the cooking is completed.

Blueberry Almond
Oatmeal, p. 81

BREAKFASTS

BLUEBERRY ALMOND OATMEAL 81

MUSHROOM SPINACH ARTICHOKE
BREAKFAST CASSEROLE 82

MAIN DISHES

BUTTERNUT SQUASH CHICKPEA STEW 83

STACKED ENCHILADA CASSEROLE 84

VEGETABLE LASAGNA 85

CHICKEN CACCIATORE 86

TURKEY CHILI 87

BEEF WITH BROCCOLI 88

DESSERTS

BAKED APPLES 89

MIXED BERRY COMPOTE 90

BLUEBERRY ALMOND OATMEAL

VEGETARIAN · GLUTEN-FREE · DAIRY-FREE

The oats in this dish are naturally gluten-free, but some varieties are processed in facilities where cross-contamination may occur. If this is a concern, look for oats labeled gluten-free. Blueberries and maple syrup round out this dish to provide a sweet taste that will keep you satisfied until lunch.

SERVES: *8*

PREP TIME: *5 minutes*

COOK TIME: *8 hours*

4 cups water

2 cups almond milk

2 cups old-fashioned rolled oats

2 cups frozen blueberries

¼ cup pure maple syrup

½ cup sliced almonds

1. Put the water, almond milk, oats, blueberries, syrup, and almonds in a slow cooker and stir.

2. Cover and cook on low for 8 hours.

3. Divide into 8 servings.

SUBSTITUTE! You can customize this recipe to fit your personal dietary needs by using nonfat milk, soy milk, or coconut milk instead of almond milk.

STORAGE: Keep individual servings in the refrigerator for up to five days.

Per serving: Calories: 184, Total Fat: 6g, Protein: 5g, Carbohydrates: 28g, Sugars: 10g, Fiber: 4g, Sodium: 92mg

MUSHROOM SPINACH ARTICHOKE BREAKFAST CASSEROLE

VEGETARIAN • GLUTEN-FREE • NUT-FREE

This breakfast casserole is packed with vegetables and eggs, both of which support weight loss. These days there is a lot of confusion about whether or not eggs are healthy. Despite sensational headlines, most people can eat one to two whole eggs per day without negative consequences. In addition to supporting weight loss, eggs provide protein and other important nutrients, making them an ideal ingredient in this recipe.

SERVES: *4*

PREP TIME: *15 minutes*

COOK TIME: *6 hours*

Nonstick cooking spray

2 tablespoons olive oil

4 ounces white or baby bella mushrooms, sliced

2 garlic cloves or 2 teaspoons jarred, minced garlic

1 (10-ounce) package frozen chopped spinach, thawed and drained

1 (14-ounce) can artichoke hearts, not marinated, drained

2 tablespoons fresh dill or 2 teaspoons dried dill

1 teaspoon salt

½ teaspoon freshly ground black pepper

1 cup nonfat milk

6 eggs

½ cup shredded Swiss cheese

1. Spray the inside of the slow cooker with cooking spray, including the bottom and sides.

2. Using the sauté setting on the slow cooker, heat the olive oil. Add the mushrooms and garlic, and cook for about 3 minutes.

3. Add the spinach, artichoke hearts, dill, salt, and pepper, stirring to mix.

4. Add the milk and the eggs. Using a fork or mixing spoon, stir to "scramble" the eggs, breaking the yolks and mixing them in with the vegetables.

5. Sprinkle the Swiss cheese on top of the mixture.

6. Cover and cook on low for 6 hours.

7. Divide into 4 servings.

SUBSTITUTE! *If you can't find frozen spinach or simply have fresh spinach on hand, use 10 ounces of fresh spinach instead. Add the fresh spinach with the mushrooms and garlic to sauté.*

Per serving: Calories: 305, Total Fat: 18g, Protein: 20g, Carbohydrates: 20g, Sugars: 6g, Fiber: 8g, Sodium: 787mg

BUTTERNUT SQUASH CHICKPEA STEW

VEGETARIAN · GLUTEN-FREE · NUT-FREE

This hearty stew is filled with nutritious ingredients that support your weight loss efforts by promoting satiety. Butternut squash is a good source of vitamin C, fiber, potassium, and beta-carotene, which gives the flesh its yellow-orange color. It supports eye health, bone health, and even proper immune function. The chickpeas are a good source of fiber, protein, and carbohydrates and have been shown to support healthy blood sugar levels and heart health.

SERVES: 6

PREP TIME: *15 minutes*

COOK TIME: *4 to 6 hours*

1 tablespoon olive oil

1 small onion, chopped

2 garlic cloves or 2 teaspoons jarred, minced garlic

1 pound fresh or frozen butternut squash, diced

1 (15½ ounce) can chickpeas, drained and rinsed

1 (8-ounce) can tomato sauce

1 teaspoon dried sage or 1 tablespoon fresh sage

1 teaspoon salt

½ teaspoon freshly ground black pepper

4 cups vegetable or chicken broth

1 pound kale, chopped

¼ cup grated Parmesan cheese, divided

1. Put the olive oil, onion, and garlic in a slow cooker on the sauté setting. Sauté for 3 to 4 minutes.

2. Add the squash, chickpeas, tomato sauce, sage, salt, and pepper.

3. Pour the broth over the mixture and stir to combine.

4. Cook on low for 6 hours or on high for 4 hours.

5. In the last 20 minutes, add the kale to the slow cooker and stir. Cover and cook for the remaining time.

6. Divide into 6 bowls and top each with 1 tablespoon of Parmesan cheese.

SUBSTITUTE! *You can adapt this recipe based on what you have on hand by using 10 ounces of fresh spinach or 10 ounces of a kale-spinach blend in place of the kale.*

STORAGE: *Store in the refrigerator for up to four days or freeze individual servings for up to six months.*

SHORTCUT! *Use precut squash from the produce or freezer section to save time.*

Per serving: Calories: 218, Total Fat: 5g, Protein: 12g, Carbohydrates: 33g, Sugars: 6g, Fiber: 7g, Sodium: 791mg

STACKED ENCHILADA CASSEROLE

VEGETARIAN · GLUTEN-FREE · NUT-FREE

Traditionally, enchiladas are rolled corn tortillas, but this recipe offers a twist by stacking them into a casserole. When making enchiladas, always use corn tortillas rather than wheat flour tortillas. Corn tortillas have about half the calories of the wheat flour tortillas of the same size and contain more fiber and fewer ingredients. You can choose either white corn or yellow corn tortillas for this dish.

SERVES: *6*

PREP TIME: *15 minutes*

COOK TIME: *4 hours*

2 (10-ounce) cans enchilada sauce, divided

12 (6-inch) corn tortillas

1 (15¼-ounce) can black beans, drained and rinsed

1 cup frozen corn or 1 (8¾-ounce) can whole-kernel corn, drained

1 teaspoon ground cumin, divided

1 teaspoon chili powder, divided

1½ cups shredded Monterey Jack cheese, divided

1. Spread ¼ cup of enchilada sauce over the bottom of a slow cooker.

2. Layer four corn tortillas over the enchilada sauce to cover the bottom of the slow cooker.

3. Layer half the black beans, half the corn, ½ teaspoon of cumin, ½ teaspoon of chili powder, and ½ cup of Monterey Jack cheese, spreading each evenly over the tortillas. Pour ¾ cup of enchilada sauce over this layer.

4. Layer four more tortillas on top. Add the remaining black beans, corn, cumin, and chili powder. Add another ½ cup of cheese and ¾ cup of enchilada sauce.

5. Layer the final four tortillas on top of the mixture.

6. Pour the remaining enchilada sauce over the tortillas and top with the remaining cheese.

7. Cover and cook on low for 4 hours. Divide into 6 servings.

SUBSTITUTE! *You can use pinto beans in place of the black beans without altering the flavor profile too much.*

STORAGE: *Store individual servings in the refrigerator for up to three days or freeze for up to one month.*

SHORTCUT! *On meal prep day, toss together the beans, corn, and spices and store in the refrigerator until assembly time. Use half of the mix for each layer.*

Per serving: Calories: 322, Total Fat: 12g, Protein: 15g, Carbohydrates: 41g, Sugars: 2g, Fiber: 8g, Sodium: 796mg

VEGETABLE LASAGNA

VEGETARIAN · NUT-FREE

Due to the cooking time and the layers in this lasagna, there is no need to cook the noodles ahead of time or buy oven-ready versions of the pasta. The liquid from the sauce, ricotta cheese, and vegetables, combined with the cooking time, will thoroughly cook the noodles.

SERVES: 6

PREP TIME: *20 minutes*

COOK TIME: *5 hours*

1 (24-ounce) jar tomato and basil pasta sauce, divided

1 (16-ounce) package whole wheat lasagna noodles

1 (15-ounce) container ricotta cheese

2 medium zucchini, sliced

1 (6-ounce) package baby spinach

1 red bell pepper, chopped

2 tablespoons fresh oregano or 2 teaspoons dried oregano, divided

1 cup shredded mozzarella cheese, divided

1. Spread ½ cup of pasta sauce evenly over the bottom of a slow cooker.

2. Place the lasagna noodles over the pasta sauce, breaking them to fit as needed.

3. Spread half of the ricotta over the noodles.

4. Layer half of the zucchini, half of the spinach, and half of the bell pepper over the ricotta cheese.

5. Sprinkle with 1 teaspoon of oregano and ⅓ cup of mozzarella cheese, then add ¾ cup of pasta sauce.

6. Make another layer of noodles, breaking them to fit.

7. Top with the remaining ricotta, zucchini, spinach, bell pepper, oregano, ⅓ cup of mozzarella cheese, and ¾ cup of pasta sauce.

8. Add a final layer of lasagna noodles and top with the remaining pasta sauce and mozzarella cheese.

9. Cover and cook on low for 5 hours.

10. Divide into 6 servings.

SUBSTITUTE! *If you're looking to cut calories or reduce fat, you can use cottage cheese in place of the ricotta cheese.*

SHORTCUT! *This can be made the day ahead. Assemble in the slow cooker, cover with foil, and store in the refrigerator for up to one day before cooking. Cook on low for 6 hours.*

Per serving: Calories: 497, Total Fat: 12g, Protein: 25g, Carbohydrates: 73g, Sugars: 11g, Fiber: 11g, Sodium: 271mg

CHICKEN CACCIATORE

GLUTEN-FREE • NUT-FREE • DAIRY-FREE

There are several ways to prepare chicken cacciatore. Some recipes don't include mushrooms and others will include red or white wine in the cooking. Other recipes include different herbs and spices, including paprika. This version features health-supporting vegetables by including mushrooms and tomatoes.

SERVES: 6

PREP TIME: 20 minutes

COOK TIME: 4 to 6 hours

1 tablespoon olive oil

8 ounces white or baby bella mushrooms, sliced

1 medium green bell pepper, sliced

1 medium yellow onion, sliced

3 garlic cloves, minced, or 3 teaspoons jarred, minced garlic

1½ pounds boneless, skinless chicken breast or chicken tenderloins

1 teaspoon salt

1 teaspoon freshly ground black pepper

2 teaspoons dried oregano

2 teaspoons dried basil

1 (28-ounce) can crushed tomatoes

1 (6-ounce) can tomato paste

2 tablespoons balsamic vinegar

Hot, cooked pasta or polenta (optional)

1. Heat the olive oil in a slow cooker on the sauté setting. Sauté the mushrooms, bell pepper, onion, and garlic for 3 to 4 minutes.

2. Add the chicken and sprinkle the salt, pepper, oregano, and basil evenly over it.

3. Pour the crushed tomatoes with their juice and the tomato paste over the chicken and vegetables.

4. Cover and cook on low for 6 hours or on high for 4 hours.

5. When it's done cooking, stir in the balsamic vinegar and let sit for 10 minutes.

6. Divide the chicken into six portions, serve over pasta or polenta (if using), and pour the sauce over the chicken.

SUBSTITUTE! *For a similar flavor profile, you can use Italian seasoning in place of the oregano and basil.*

STORAGE: *Store in the refrigerator for up to four days. Freeze individual servings without pasta for up to three months.*

SHORTCUT! *Skip the sauté step and add all the ingredients, except the balsamic vinegar, to the cooking pot. Continue as directed.*

Per serving: Calories: 246, Total Fat: 4g, Protein: 32g, Carbohydrates: 21g, Sugars: 13g, Fiber: 6g, Sodium: 647mg

TURKEY CHILI

GLUTEN-FREE · NUT-FREE

People often think of turkey only for year-end holiday meals, but it is a healthy lean protein you can eat year-round. Whether you want to decrease your red-meat intake or you're looking for an alternative to chicken, turkey is an excellent option for many soups, stews, and chilis.

SERVES: *4*

PREP TIME: *20 minutes*

COOK TIME: *4 to 6 hours*

1 small onion, diced

1 pound lean ground turkey

3 cups tomato juice or vegetable juice

2 (15½-ounce) cans kidney beans, drained and rinsed

1 (14½-ounce) can diced tomatoes

1 red bell pepper, diced

2 tablespoons chili powder

1 teaspoon salt

½ teaspoon freshly ground black pepper

½ cup shredded Cheddar cheese, divided

1. Put the onions in a slow cooker on the sauté or browning setting. Cook for 1 to 2 minutes. Add the turkey and brown for 4 to 6 minutes, stirring to break it up. The turkey does not need to be fully cooked.

2. Add the tomato juice, kidney beans, diced tomatoes with their juice, bell pepper, chili powder, salt, and pepper. Stir to combine the mixture.

3. Cover and cook on low heat for 6 hours or on high heat for 4 hours.

4. Divide into 4 bowls and top each with 2 tablespoons of cheese.

SUBSTITUTE! *If you don't have kidney beans on hand, you can use two cans of pinto beans or white beans instead.*

STORAGE: *Store in the refrigerator for up to three days or in the freezer (without the cheese) for up to six months.*

SHORTCUT! *If your slow cooker has no sauté feature to brown the onion and meat, simply break up the turkey with your hands or a spoon before adding the rest of the ingredients.*

Per serving: Calories: 466, Total Fat: 15g, Protein: 41g, Carbohydrates: 48g, Sugars: 12g, Fiber: 14g, Sodium: 1,098mg

BEEF WITH BROCCOLI

NUT-FREE • DAIRY-FREE

Combining beef and broccoli in this dish provides a nice metabolism-friendly balance. Between the high protein value of the beef and the fiber and nutrients in the broccoli, you're not only supporting your weight loss efforts but your overall digestive health as well. When preparing dishes in the slow cooker, you can use tougher, less expensive cuts of meat since the longer cooking method helps make the meat more tender.

SERVES: *4*

PREP TIME: *15 minutes*

COOK TIME: *4 hours*

1 pound beef tenderloin strips

1 cup low-sodium beef broth

¼ cup low-sodium soy sauce

2 tablespoons brown sugar

2 tablespoons sesame oil

1 tablespoon red pepper flakes (optional)

2 garlic cloves, minced, or 2 teaspoons jarred, minced garlic

1 pound broccoli florets

Hot, cooked rice (optional)

1. Combine the beef, broth, soy sauce, brown sugar, sesame oil, red pepper flakes, and garlic in a slow cooker.

2. Cook on low for 4 hours.

3. In the last 20 minutes, add in the broccoli and stir.

4. Cover and finish cooking.

5. Divide into 4 portions and serve with the rice (if using).

SUBSTITUTE! *To make this dish gluten-free, substitute tamari sauce for soy sauce.*

STORAGE: *Store in the refrigerator for up to three days.*

Per serving: Calories: 303, Total Fat: 15g, Protein: 30g, Carbohydrates: 14g, Sugars: 8g, Fiber: 3g, Sodium: 826mg

BAKED APPLES

VEGETARIAN • VEGAN • GLUTEN-FREE • DAIRY-FREE

There are many varieties of apples, and some are better for baking than others. The green Granny Smith apple is popular, as are the red Honeycrisp, Braeburn, and Gala. Choose your favorite variety or even do a mix for this dessert. Eat the finished dish on its own or use it as a topping for oatmeal, yogurt, or cottage cheese.

SERVES: *8*

PREP TIME: *10 minutes*

COOK TIME: *2 to 4 hours*

2 pounds Granny Smith apples, sliced and cored

½ cup chopped walnuts

½ cup pure maple syrup

1 teaspoon cinnamon

1. Layer the apples in the bottom of a slow cooker.

2. Sprinkle the walnuts over the apples.

3. Pour the maple syrup over the apples and walnuts.

4. Sprinkle the cinnamon over the mixture.

5. Cover and cook on low for 2 to 4 hours. Two hours yields crisper apples while four hours yields much softer apples.

6. Divide into 8 portions.

STORAGE: *If not eaten warm, store in the refrigerator for up to a week.*

Per serving: Calories: 123, Total Fat: 4g, Protein: 1g, Carbohydrates: 22g, Sugars: 18g, Fiber: 2g, Sodium: 2mg

MIXED BERRY COMPOTE

VEGETARIAN · VEGAN · GLUTEN-FREE · NUT-FREE · DAIRY-FREE

Berries are loaded with nutrients that can reduce the risk of cancer and heart disease. They are also high in fiber, which supports a healthy digestive system. Choose your favorite berries or seasonal fruit to make your own unique fruit dessert, mix-in, or topping with this recipe. One pound of fruit will make about two cups, so this recipe is simple to scale. This is great to use when there is a seasonal crop of fruit that may go bad before you can eat it.

SERVES: *12*

PREP TIME: *10 minutes*

COOK TIME: *2 to 3 hours*

1 pound (about 2 cups) blueberries, fresh or frozen

1 pound (about 2 cups) raspberries, fresh or frozen

1 pound (about 2 cups) strawberries, fresh or frozen

Juice of 1 orange

1 teaspoon ground cinnamon

1. If using fresh fruit remove the stems from the strawberries.

2. Put the blueberries, raspberries, and strawberries in a slow cooker.

3. Pour the orange juice over the berries.

4. Sprinkle with the cinnamon.

5. Cover and cook on low for 2 hours if using fresh berries, or for 3 hours if using frozen berries.

6. Divide into 12 servings and serve warm.

SUBSTITUTE! *This recipe works with any seasonal fresh fruit such as apricots, cherries, nectarines, peaches, plums, and more.*

STORAGE: *Store in the refrigerator for up to two weeks.*

Per serving: Calories: 57, Total Fat: 1g, Protein: 1g, Carbohydrates: 14g, Sugars: 8g, Fiber: 4g, Sodium: 1mg

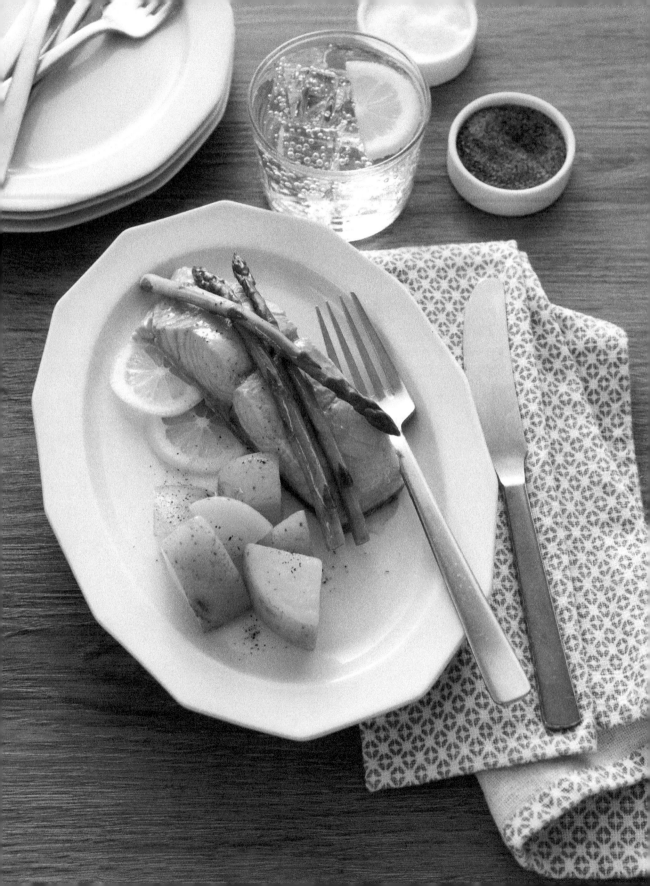

ELECTRIC PRESSURE COOKER

With a variety of makes and models of electric pressure cookers on the market, it's always a good idea to read the instructions for how to operate yours first.

Some of these recipes use a sauté feature for certain ingredients before switching to the pressure cooker mode, so make sure you know how to use that feature. Also note that cooking times in the following recipes are listed with an additional "plus pressure time." While the actual cooking time is listed, the amount of time it takes for your model to become fully pressurized will vary.

Here are my best tips for using a pressure cooker:

- Ensure that the gasket is in place. Otherwise, the food will be steamed, not pressure-cooked.

- Ensure that the steam release handle is closed at the start of the cycle.

- Use caution when releasing the steam at the end of cooking time, as it can cause burns.

- If you are unable to open the lid after the cycle is complete and you have opened the steam release, double-check that the valve itself is also released.

Salmon with Potatoes and Asparagus, p. 102

QUINOA BREAKFAST BOWLS WITH APPLES AND PEANUT BUTTER

VEGAN • VEGETARIAN • GLUTEN-FREE • DAIRY-FREE • 30 MINUTES OR LESS

I chose quinoa (pronounced KEEN-wah) for this dish due to its amazing nutritional profile. It's one of the few plant foods that is also considered a complete protein, which means it has all nine of the protein-building amino acids humans need in a single food. This protein-packed dish promotes satiety, which aids in your weight loss efforts, while also providing the natural sweetness of apples and honey.

SERVES: *4*

PREP TIME: *5 minutes*

COOK TIME: *2 minutes*

(plus pressure time)

1 cup quinoa

1 cup water

2 tablespoons peanut butter

2 Granny Smith apples, diced

1 tablespoon honey

½ cup nonfat milk or nut milk (optional), divided

1. In a strainer, rinse the quinoa to remove the bitter coating.

2. In a pressure cooker, combine the quinoa, water, peanut butter, and apples.

3. Cover and seal, ensuring that the vent is closed.

4. Cook for 2 minutes.

5. When it's done cooking, allow the steam to vent.

6. Remove the lid, add the honey, and stir well.

7. Divide into 4 servings and add the milk (if using).

SUBSTITUTE! *If you're looking to increase your dietary fiber or consume more healthy fats, consider using almond butter in place of the peanut butter.*

STORAGE: *This dish may be made ahead and stored in the refrigerator for up to one week. When you're ready to eat it, you can reheat in the microwave or serve it cold.*

Per serving: Calories: 277, Total Fat: 7g, Protein: 8g, Carbohydrates: 49g, Sugars: 17g, Fiber: 6g, Sodium: 40mg

SPINACH AND TOMATO EGG BREAKFAST

VEGETARIAN • GLUTEN-FREE • NUT-FREE • 30 MINUTES OR LESS

Choline is a nutrient that humans can only get from food. It is important for healthy brain development, muscle movement, and nerve function. One of the best sources of this nutrient is eggs. Choosing eggs in moderation, a few times a week, is fine and does not appear to have a negative impact on heart health as it once was believed. When combined with the fresh spinach and tomatoes, this breakfast dish packs a nutritional punch, complete with many vitamins and minerals you need to feel energized during the day.

SERVES: *4*

PREP TIME: *10 minutes*

COOK TIME: *15 minutes*

(plus pressure time)

1 cup water

1 teaspoon olive oil

6 large eggs

½ cup nonfat milk

1 cup fresh spinach, chopped

1 cup halved grape or cherry tomatoes

½ teaspoon dried basil

½ teaspoon dried oregano

¼ cup (1 ounce) feta cheese, crumbled

1. In a pressure cooker, pour in the water and put a metal trivet on the bottom.

2. Use the oil to grease a round baking pan, such as a cake or pie pan, then add the eggs and scramble them with a fork.

3. Add the milk, spinach, tomatoes, basil, and oregano. Stir to mix and top with the feta.

4. Set the pan in the pot on the trivet.

5. Cover and seal, checking that the vent is closed, and set to pressure cook for 15 minutes.

6. When it's done cooking, allow the steam to vent.

7. Divide into 4 servings and serve.

SUBSTITUTE! *If you don't like the crumbly texture or taste of feta, mozzarella cheese is a great alternative.*

STORAGE: *Store in the refrigerator for up to three days.*

SHORTCUT! *If you're running short on time or don't have eggs on hand, you can use ¾ cup liquid eggs from a carton instead.*

Per serving: Calories: 164, Total Fat: 11g, Protein: 12g, Carbohydrates: 5g, Sugars: 4g, Fiber: 1g, Sodium: 234mg

FRENCH TOAST CASSEROLE

VEGETARIAN · NUT-FREE

This delicious recipe gives you the taste of French toast without the added calories of frying. Many types of bread can be used for French toast, including sourdough or challah. For best results, use day-old bread or bread that is a bit dried out. You can also cut up the bread the day before making this dish to help dry it out.

SERVES: 6

PREP TIME: *10 minutes*

COOK TIME: *25 minutes*

(plus pressure time)

1 cup water

Nonstick cooking spray

1 (16-ounce) loaf cinnamon raisin bread, cut into 1-inch cubes

1 cup nonfat milk

6 large eggs

1. In a pressure cooker, pour in the water and put a metal trivet on the bottom.

2. Spray the inside of an oven-proof glass bowl with cooking spray and put it inside the pressure cooker.

3. Put the bread in the bowl.

4. In a 2- or 4-cup liquid measuring cup, combine the milk and eggs. With a fork, mix to break up the egg yolks and blend in with the milk.

5. Pour the egg and milk mixture over the cubed bread.

6. Cover and seal, checking that the vent is closed, and set to pressure cook for 25 minutes.

7. When it's done cooking, allow the steam to vent.

8. Divide into 6 servings.

SUBSTITUTE! *If you don't have cinnamon raisin bread, simply add 1 teaspoon of cinnamon and ¼ cup of raisins to the bowl with your bread of choice before pouring the milk and egg mixture over the bread.*

STORAGE: *Allow casserole to cool completely, then store in the refrigerator for up to three days.*

Per serving: Calories: 299, Total Fat: 9g, Protein: 12g, Carbohydrates: 43g, Sugars: 19g, Fiber: 2g, Sodium: 339mg

CAULIFLOWER POTATO SOUP

VEGETARIAN · GLUTEN-FREE · NUT-FREE · 30 MINUTES OR LESS

This recipe is a lighter version of the classic baked potato soup, using cauliflower. While it contains fewer calories than the traditional recipe, it still has that baked potato flavor you know and love. For a smoother consistency, you can use an immersion blender to purée the vegetables after cooking. For a chunkier soup, simply grab a potato masher. Once you top it with the cheese and yogurt, your family will never guess this is a healthy take on a beloved classic.

SERVES: *4*

PREP TIME: *15 minutes*

COOK TIME: *10 minutes*
(plus pressure time)

1½ pounds russet potatoes, diced (peeled, optional)

1 pound fresh cauliflower florets

3 cups low-sodium vegetable broth or chicken broth

½ cup diced yellow onion

4 cloves garlic or 1 tablespoon jarred, minced garlic

1 teaspoon dried thyme

1 cup nonfat milk

¼ cup shredded Cheddar cheese, divided

¼ cup plain, fat-free Greek yogurt, divided

1. In a pressure cooker, put the potatoes, cauliflower, broth, onion, garlic, and thyme.

2. Cover and cook for 10 minutes.

3. When it's done cooking, allow the steam to vent.

4. Remove the lid and stir in the milk.

5. Using a masher, mash the vegetables until a thick soup forms.

6. Divide into 4 bowls and top each with 1 tablespoon cheese and 1 tablespoon yogurt.

SUBSTITUTE! *If you don't have fresh cauliflower on hand, you can use frozen cauliflower instead. You can also use unpeeled red potatoes in place of the russet potatoes.*

STORAGE: *Store in the refrigerator (without the cheese and yogurt) for up to four days. Add the cheese and yogurt after reheating.*

Per serving: Calories: 228, Total Fat: 3g, Protein: 12g, Carbohydrates: 40g, Sugars: 9g, Fiber: 7g, Sodium: 174mg

LENTIL SPINACH SOUP

VEGETARIAN · VEGAN · GLUTEN-FREE · NUT-FREE · DAIRY-FREE

Lentils come in a variety of colors, including green, brown, yellow, and red. Some hold up to high pressure better than others, so this recipe calls for green or brown lentils. Lentils are a budget-friendly, plant-based protein. They're also high in complex carbohydrates that support healthy metabolism. This recipe pairs lentils with spinach, which is low in calories and high in water and fiber, to help maximize weight loss.

SERVES: *4*

PREP TIME: *10 minutes*

COOK TIME: *25 minutes*

(plus pressure time)

1 cup diced carrots

½ cup diced onions

½ cup diced celery

3 garlic cloves, crushed, or 1 tablespoon jarred, minced garlic

1¼ cups dried green or brown lentils

1 teaspoon ground cumin

1 teaspoon coriander

½ teaspoon freshly ground black pepper

4 cups low-sodium vegetable broth

6 ounces fresh spinach, chopped

¼ cup grated Parmesan cheese, divided (optional)

1. Using the sauté setting on a pressure cooker, cook the carrots, onions, and celery for 4 minutes.

2. Add the garlic and sauté for 1 minute.

3. Add the lentils, cumin, coriander, pepper, and broth.

4. Stop the sauté setting, cover, and set the pressure cooker setting on high for 15 minutes.

5. When it's done cooking, let it sit for 10 minutes without opening or releasing the pressure valve. After 10 minutes, open the valve to ensure that any remaining pressure is released.

6. Open the lid and add the spinach, stirring to wilt.

7. Divide into 4 servings and top each with 1 tablespoon of Parmesan cheese (if using).

SUBSTITUTE! *Depending on what you have on hand, you can use 10 ounces of frozen spinach instead of fresh. Just add the frozen spinach to the pressure cooker pot with the lentils and broth.*

STORAGE: *Store in the refrigerator for up to three days or in the freezer for up to six months.*

Per serving: Calories: 238, Total Fat: 1g, Protein: 18g, Carbohydrates: 39g, Sugars: 2g, Fiber: 8g, Sodium: 135mg

MACARONI AND CHEESE WITH BROCCOLI

VEGETARIAN · NUT-FREE

Making a classic comfort food dish like macaroni and cheese a bit healthier is simple with the addition of some vegetables. The classic combination of broccoli and cheese is a delicious way to enjoy more veggies. This recipe makes a lot and may easily be cut in half.

SERVES: *8*

PREP TIME: *10 minutes*

COOK TIME: *10 minutes*
(plus pressure time)

16 ounces whole wheat elbow macaroni or similar pasta, such as shells or rotini

4 cups low-sodium vegetable broth

1 teaspoon garlic powder

1 teaspoon dry mustard

1 cup nonfat milk

1½ cups shredded, sharp Cheddar cheese

2 tablespoons Neufchâtel cheese

3 cups broccoli florets

1. In a pressure cooker, put the pasta, broth, garlic powder, and mustard.

2. Cover and seal, ensuring that the vent is closed.

3. Set to pressure cook on high for 4 minutes.

4. When it's done cooking, allow the steam to vent.

5. Remove the lid and add the milk, cheddar cheese, and Neufchâtel cheese. Stir to mix and allow the cheeses to melt.

6. Add the broccoli and mix. Cover and let sit for 5 minutes.

7. Divide into 8 individual servings.

SUBSTITUTE! *Depending on your taste preferences or dietary needs, you can substitute any fresh vegetables, such as carrots, tomatoes or cauliflower, for the broccoli. For example, if you want more antioxidant-rich vegetables in your diet, choose carrots or tomatoes. For more fiber, stick with the broccoli or choose cauliflower.*

STORAGE: *Store in the refrigerator for up to four days.*

Per serving: Calories: 338, Total Fat: 9g, Protein: 16g, Carbohydrates: 47g, Sugars: 4g, Fiber: 3g, Sodium: 211mg

MUSHROOM RISOTTO

VEGETARIAN · GLUTEN-FREE · NUT-FREE

Traditionally, risotto requires monitoring and constant stirring for 20 to 30 minutes to get its creamy texture. The pressure cooker lets you skip that labor-intensive activity with the same result. Arborio rice, which is a short-grain rice, provides essential vitamins along with the iron and protein you need while losing weight.

SERVES: *4*

PREP TIME: *10 minutes*

COOK TIME: *15 minutes*

(plus pressure time)

2 tablespoons olive oil

½ cup onions, diced

8 ounces white or baby bella mushrooms, sliced

2 garlic cloves or 2 teaspoons jarred, minced garlic

2 cups low-sodium vegetable broth

1 cup arborio rice

1 teaspoon dried thyme

10 ounces fresh spinach, chopped

¼ cup grated Parmesan cheese, divided

1. Using the sauté setting on a pressure cooker, heat the oil. Add the onion, mushrooms, and garlic.

2. Sauté for 7 minutes.

3. Add the broth, rice, and thyme, and stir.

4. Stop the sauté setting, cover, and start the pressure cooker setting for 6 minutes.

5. When it's done cooking, release the pressure and remove the lid.

6. Immediately add the spinach, stirring to wilt.

7. Divide into 4 servings and top each with 1 tablespoon of Parmesan cheese.

SUBSTITUTE! *For a more nutrient-dense meal, swap the spinach for a leafy green blend such as kale and spinach. If you're looking to stay more hydrated, choose arugula, which contains 90 percent water, in place of the spinach.*

STORAGE: *Store in the refrigerator for up to four days.*

Per serving: Calories: 301, Total Fat: 9g, Protein: 10g, Carbohydrates: 46g, Sugars: 2g, Fiber: 4g, Sodium: 164mg

SALMON WITH POTATOES AND ASPARAGUS

GLUTEN-FREE • NUT-FREE • DAIRY-FREE • 30 MINUTES OR LESS

This dish makes the most of ingredients you already have. Frozen salmon will keep in the freezer for about four months, meaning it's easy to keep on hand to cut on a regular basis. As a bonus, this dish does not require the salmon be defrosted—just put the frozen fillets in the pressure cooker pot to save time. Salmon, whether wild-caught or farmed, is an excellent source of omega-3 fats, which many people need to increase in their diet.

SERVES: *4*

PREP TIME: *10 minutes*

COOK TIME: *10 minutes*

(plus pressure time)

1 cup low-sodium vegetable or chicken broth

1 pound Yukon gold potatoes, cut into 2-inch pieces

1 pound frozen salmon fillets

2 teaspoons garlic powder

2 tablespoons lemon juice

1 pound fresh asparagus, trimmed

1. Pour the broth into a pressure cooker.

2. Add the potatoes, spreading them out evenly over the bottom of the pot.

3. Layer the frozen salmon, skin-side down, over the potatoes.

4. Top with the garlic powder and lemon juice.

5. Put the asparagus in an even layer over the salmon.

6. Cover and seal the pressure cooker, ensuring that the vent is closed.

7. Cook on high for 3 minutes.

8. When it's done cooking, let it sit for 5 minutes, then allow the steam to vent.

9. Divide into 4 servings.

SUBSTITUTE! *For a more high-fiber dish, consider using fresh broccoli florets or Brussels sprouts in place of the asparagus.*

SHORTCUT! *To save time, you can skip cutting the potatoes by using fingerling potatoes instead of Yukon gold potatoes.*

Per serving: Calories: 247, Total Fat: 5g, Protein: 29g, Carbohydrates: 24g, Sugars: 4g, Fiber: 5g, Sodium: 277mg

SHRIMP BOIL

GLUTEN-FREE • NUT-FREE • DAIRY-FREE

A traditional seafood boil is a social event in which various types of shellfish are boiled with corn, potatoes, and other vegetables in a large pot. Ingredients often vary by region. After the water is drained, the pot of food is spread across a tray or table covered with butcher paper and eaten without the use of dishes or utensils. Enjoy this version with a lot less time, minimal effort, and, most important, far less mess.

SERVES: *6*

PREP TIME: *10 minutes*

COOK TIME: *30 minutes*

1 cup low-sodium chicken broth or water

1 tablespoon Old Bay Seasoning

1 medium Vidalia onion, cut into 8 pieces

6 garlic cloves, crushed, or 2 tablespoons jarred, minced garlic

6 frozen half-ear corn on the cob

6 ounces Cajun-style andouille sausage

1½ pounds large frozen shrimp, shell on

1. Put the broth or water, seasoning, onion, garlic, corn, sausage, and shrimp in a pressure cooker.

2. Put the lid on and seal, ensuring that the vent is closed.

3. Cook on high for 0 (zero) minutes.

4. Set a secondary timer for 30 minutes.

5. At the end of the 30 minutes, even if the pressure is not completely done, cancel or stop the cycle, release the pressure, and remove the lid.

6. Divide the ingredients evenly among 6 servings.

SUBSTITUTE! *For a meatier dish, use crawfish instead of the shrimp.*

STORAGE: *Store any leftovers in the refrigerator for up to three days.*

Per serving: Calories: 294, Total Fat: 8g, Protein: 36g, Carbohydrates: 19g, Sugars: 4g, Fiber: 3g, Sodium: 689mg

SWEET AND SOUR CHICKEN

GLUTEN-FREE • NUT-FREE • DAIRY-FREE

When many people think of sweet and sour sauce, they imagine the bright red sauce in Chinese takeout. Generally, sweet and sour sauce is not red, though it may have a slight pink hue from ketchup. By combining pineapples, honey, and tomato paste, you can still enjoy the sweet flavor this dish is known for without the added sugar.

SERVES: *4*

PREP TIME: *10 minutes*

COOK TIME: *15 minutes*

(plus pressure time)

1 tablespoon olive oil

1 pound boneless, skinless chicken breast, cut into 1-inch pieces

1 (20-ounce) can pineapple chunks

2 garlic cloves, crushed, or 2 teaspoons jarred, minced garlic

1 (6-ounce) can tomato paste

2 tablespoons rice vinegar

1 tablespoon honey or brown sugar

1 red bell pepper, sliced

1 green bell pepper, sliced

Hot, cooked rice (optional)

1. Using the sauté setting on a pressure cooker, heat the oil. Sauté the chicken for 2 to 3 minutes, or until brown. (Note that the chicken will not be fully cooked.)

2. Drain ½ cup of pineapple juice from the can into a 2-cup measuring cup. Discard the remaining juice.

3. Put the garlic and pineapple chunks in the pressure cooker pot.

4. Add the tomato paste, rice vinegar, and honey to the pineapple juice and stir to mix.

5. Pour the mixture over the chicken and pineapple in the pot.

6. Stop the sauté setting, cover, and start the pressure cooker setting for 5 minutes.

7. When it's done cooking, release the pressure and remove the lid.

8. Add the bell peppers to the pot and replace the lid. Let sit for 5 minutes.

9. Stir and divide into 4 servings. Serve with the rice (if using).

SUBSTITUTE! *For a slightly different flavor profile, use pork tenderloin, cut into 1-inch pieces, in place of the chicken.*

STORAGE: *Store in the refrigerator for up to four days.*

SHORTCUT! *To cut down on time and cleanup, use 10 ounces frozen bell pepper and onion blend for the fresh bell peppers.*

Per serving: Calories: 303, Total Fat: 7g, Protein: 27g, Carbohydrates: 35g, Sugars: 26g, Fiber: 5g, Sodium: 103mg

TURKEY CHILI WITH WHITE BEANS

GLUTEN-FREE • NUT-FREE

This chili supports your weight loss efforts by incorporating turkey, which contains about half the calories of a red meat. In addition, cannellini beans (also known as white kidney beans) are full of health-promoting minerals such as folate and magnesium. They've even been shown to support healthy blood sugar levels. This dish is rounded out with avocado, one of the best sources of healthy monounsaturated fatty acid. You'll feel like you're indulging while eating a meal designed to support your overall health and waistline.

SERVES: *4*

PREP TIME: *10 minutes*

COOK TIME: *30 minutes*
(plus pressure time)

1 tablespoon olive oil

1 cup yellow onion, chopped

1 medium Anaheim pepper, diced (about ½ cup)

1 pound lean ground turkey breast

1 (15½-ounce) can cannellini beans, drained and rinsed

1 (14½-ounce) can diced tomatoes

2 cups low-sodium chicken broth

2 tablespoons chili powder

1 teaspoon ground cumin

1 teaspoon coriander

½ teaspoon freshly ground black pepper

¼ cup pepper Jack cheese, divided

1 medium avocado, quartered

1. Using the sauté setting on a pressure cooker, heat the oil.

2. Add the onion and pepper and sauté for 3 to 4 minutes.

3. Add the turkey and cook for 5 minutes, breaking up the meat.

4. Add the beans, tomatoes with their juice, broth, chili powder, cumin, coriander, and pepper to the pot.

5. Stop the sauté setting, cover, and start the pressure cooker setting for 18 minutes.

6. When it's done cooking, release the pressure and remove the lid.

7. Stir to mix and divide into 4 servings. Top each with 1 tablespoon of cheese and ¼ avocado.

STORAGE: *Store in the refrigerator for up to four days or freeze for up to six months without the cheese and avocado.*

SHORTCUT! *To save time, use 2 (4-ounce) cans of green chilies in place of the diced Anaheim pepper.*

Per serving: Calories: 385, Total Fat: 15g, Protein: 37g, Carbohydrates: 29g, Sugars: 5g, Fiber: 11g, Sodium: 192mg

GROUND BEEF TACOS

NUT-FREE · DAIRY-FREE

In this family-friendly recipe, you'll use a pressure cooker to make seasoned taco meat. While the meat is cooking, set up the rest of the meal as an assembly line and let your family make their own tacos. Buy the small, street taco–size tortillas so that each serving will be two tacos.

SERVES: *4*

PREP TIME: *10 minutes*

COOK TIME: *15 minutes*

(plus pressure time)

1 pound lean ground beef

½ cup chopped onion

½ cup water

1 garlic clove, crushed,
   or 1 teaspoon jarred,
   minced garlic

1 tablespoon chili powder

1 teaspoon ground cumin

½ teaspoon salt

8 (6-inch) tortillas

½ cup shredded Cheddar
   cheese, divided

1 cup diced tomatoes,
   divided

½ cup shredded romaine
   lettuce, divided

½ cup jarred, chunky
   salsa, divided

¼ cup plain, fat-free Greek
   yogurt, divided

1. Using the sauté setting on a pressure cooker, brown the ground beef and onion for about 5 minutes, breaking up the meat. The meat will still be a little pink. Stop the sauté setting and drain any fat from the pot.

2. Add the water, garlic, chili powder, cumin, and salt.

3. Cover and set the pressure cooker on high for 5 minutes.

4. When it's done cooking, let it sit for 5 minutes before releasing the pressure.

5. Remove the lid and stir.

6. Top each tortilla with about one-eighth of the meat mixture.

7. Top each taco with 1 tablespoon of cheese, 2 tablespoons of diced tomatoes, 1 tablespoon of lettuce, 1 tablespoon of salsa, and ½ tablespoon of yogurt.

SUBSTITUTE! *Cut a few calories by making taco bowls. Just skip the tortilla and assemble the ingredients in a bowl.*

SHORTCUT! *If you're using frozen ground beef, instead of following step 1, put the beef in the pressure cooker with ½ cup of water. Cover and pressure cook set on high for 10 minutes (plus pressure time). Release the steam. Start the sauté setting and add the onion, garlic, chili powder, cumin, and salt. Sauté for 5 minutes, then proceed with the recipe.*

Per serving: Calories: 446, Total Fat: 18g, Protein: 32g, Carbohydrates: 40g, Sugars: 4g, Fiber: 4g, Sodium: 1,003mg

SPAGHETTI WITH GROUND BEEF AND VEGETABLES

NUT-FREE · DAIRY-FREE

The vegetables in this spaghetti sauce add nutrients and fiber to a classic dish and increase the number of servings, so you can feed a few more people or have leftovers. Since the zucchini and carrots are shredded, they don't overwhelm the comforting meat sauce.

SERVES: 6

PREP TIME: *10 minutes*

COOK TIME: *20 minutes*

(plus pressure time)

1 pound lean ground beef

½ cup sliced mushrooms

½ cup shredded zucchini

½ cup shredded carrots

3½ cups water

1 (16-ounce) package whole wheat spaghetti

1 (24-ounce) jar marinara sauce, no-sugar-added

1. Using the sauté setting on a pressure cooker, cook the ground beef and mushrooms for about 5 minutes, breaking up the meat until browned. Stop the sauté setting and drain any fat from the pot.

2. Add the zucchini, carrots, and water to the meat mixture and stir to combine.

3. Break the spaghetti in half and layer in a crisscross pattern over the meat and vegetables. Use a spoon to push the pasta down into the liquid as much as possible.

4. Pour the marinara sauce over the spaghetti and meat.

5. Cover and set the pressure cooker on high for 5 minutes.

6. When it's done cooking, let it sit for 5 minutes before releasing the pressure.

7. Remove the lid and stir.

8. Let it rest for 5 minutes, then divide it into 6 servings.

SUBSTITUTE! *You can substitute any shredded vegetables for the carrots and zucchini, depending on your nutritional goals and preferences. Shredded butternut squash is a great option if you don't have zucchini on hand. It has a sweet, slightly nutty taste and supports weight loss, heart health, and more.*

STORAGE: *Store in the refrigerator for up to four days.*

Per serving: Calories: 299, Total Fat: 7g, Protein: 22g, Carbohydrates: 39g, Sugars: 6g, Fiber: 2g, Sodium: 354mg

POACHED PEARS

VEGETARIAN • GLUTEN-FREE • DAIRY-FREE • 30 MINUTES OR LESS

Poached pears are often made with white wine, red wine, or port. But using grape juice will provide similar heart health benefits without the added calories of alcohol. Choose pears that are ripe and firm (but not hard). There are dozens of different varieties, but the best pears for this recipe are Anjou, Bartlett, or Bosc, which keep their shape when cooking.

SERVES: *6*

PREP TIME: *10 minutes*

COOK TIME: *8 minutes*

(plus pressure time)

4 cups water

2 cups purple or white grape juice, 100% juice

3 tablespoons honey

1 tablespoon lemon juice

1 teaspoon cinnamon

6 ripe pears, peeled

1. In a pressure cooker, put the water, grape juice, honey, lemon juice, and cinnamon.

2. Place the pears evenly, standing up, in the bottom of the pot.

3. Cover and set the pressure cooker for 8 minutes.

4. When it's done cooking, release the pressure and remove the lid.

5. Serve each pear with some of the cooking liquid.

SUBSTITUTE! *For a tart kick, replace the grape juice with pomegranate juice.*

STORAGE: *Store in the refrigerator for up to one week.*

SHORTCUT! *Skip peeling the pears and, after cooking, let sit for 5 minutes before releasing the pressure.*

Per serving: Calories: 186, Total Fat: 0g, Protein: 1g, Carbohydrates: 48g, Sugars: 37g, Fiber: 7g, Sodium: 4mg

RICE PUDDING

VEGETARIAN · VEGAN · GLUTEN-FREE · DAIRY-FREE · 30 MINUTES OR LESS

Rice pudding is a versatile dish: It can be made many different ways and be served warm or cold. The basic recipe is cooked rice, milk, and sugar with some spices. This healthy twist cuts back on the added sugar by using honey instead, and the coconut milk and almonds provide a different flavor profile.

SERVES: 6

PREP TIME: *10 minutes*

COOK TIME: *25 minutes*

(plus pressure time)

1½ cups coconut milk

1½ cups water

½ cup arborio rice

3 tablespoons honey

¼ cup raisins

¼ cup slivered almonds

½ teaspoon ground cinnamon

½ teaspoon vanilla extract

1. In a pressure cooker, mix the coconut milk, water, rice, honey, raisins, almonds, and cinnamon.

2. Cover and set the pressure cooker for 10 minutes.

3. When it's done cooking, let it sit for 10 minutes.

4. Release the pressure, remove the lid, and allow to cool for 3 minutes. Stir in the vanilla.

5. Divide into 6 servings and serve warm.

SUBSTITUTE! *If you have it on hand, you can use almond or soy milk in place of the coconut milk. Make sure not to use regular milk, since it will scald and burn. For an even nuttier flavor, you can use brown rice instead of arborio rice.*

STORAGE: *If not serving warm, allow to cool for 30 minutes and store in the refrigerator for up to two days.*

Per serving: Calories: 269, Total Fat: 16g, Protein: 4g, Carbohydrates: 30g, Sugars: 14g, Fiber: 3g, Sodium: 11mg

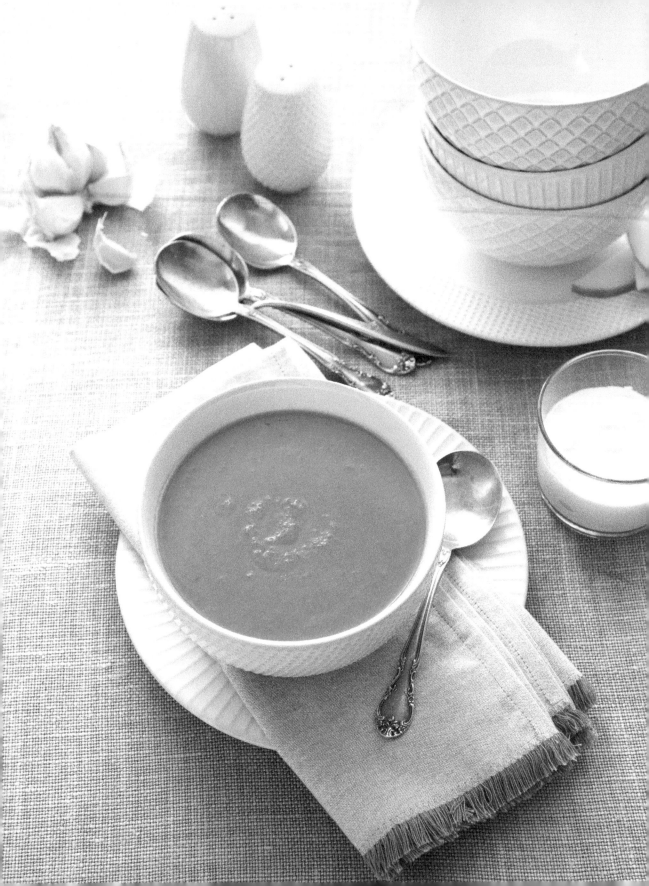

CHAPTER 7

SOUP POT

Unless otherwise stated, recipes use a 6- to 8-quart soup pot. Not all recipes will require the use of lids, but it is something you need to keep your dishes warm.

When leaving soup pots unattended, always be sure that the handle is turned in and the burner is set on low to simmer. Simmering involves lower heat and smaller bubbles, while boiling involves higher heat with larger bubbles. It is common to want to boil rather than simmer to cook food faster, but allowing your dish to simmer slowly will provide the best flavors. It will be well worth the wait!

Carrot Apple Soup
with Turmeric, p. 115

BREAKFASTS

MIXED BERRY SOUP 113

TOMATO AND SPINACH BREAKFAST STEW 114

MAIN DISHES

CARROT APPLE SOUP WITH TURMERIC 115

LENTIL SOUP WITH COLLARD GREENS 116

TORTELLINI SOUP WITH CHICKPEAS 117

PASTA E FAGIOLI 118

CHICKEN AND DUMPLINGS 119

CHICKEN PESTO SOUP 120

BEEF STEW 121

DESSERT

CHOCOLATE OAT NUT DESSERT DROPS 122

MIXED BERRY SOUP

VEGETARIAN · GLUTEN-FREE · NUT-FREE

This mixed berry soup can be used as a topping for various breakfast dishes such as oatmeal or cream of wheat. You can also simply shake it with a cup of milk to make a quick and easy smoothie without the blender. This is a good recipe to use up berries that are about to be overripe or to take advantage of peak berry seasons.

SERVES: 6

PREP TIME: 5 minutes

COOK TIME: 10 minutes

3 cups fresh berries of choice

1½ cups white or purple grape juice, 100% juice

1 tablespoon lemon juice

1 teaspoon ground cinnamon

1 teaspoon vanilla extract

1 (24-ounce) container plain, fat-free Greek yogurt

1. Put the berries in a soup pot.

2. Add the grape juice, lemon juice, and cinnamon, stirring to mix.

3. Put the pot over medium heat and bring to a boil. Reduce the heat to low and simmer for 10 minutes.

4. Remove from the heat, add the vanilla, and stir to combine.

5. Let cool, then stir in the yogurt.

6. Divide into 6 servings.

SUBSTITUTE! *If you're making this dish after peak berry season, you can use a 16-ounce bag of no-sugar-added frozen berries instead of fresh berries.*

STORAGE: *Store in the refrigerator for up to one week.*

Per serving: Calories: 121, Total Fat: 0g, Protein: 12g, Carbohydrates: 18g, Sugars: 13g, Fiber: 2g, Sodium: 2mg

TOMATO AND SPINACH
BREAKFAST STEW

VEGETARIAN · GLUTEN-FREE · NUT-FREE · 30 MINUTES OR LESS

Start your day with this breakfast vegetable stew. Each serving provides nearly two cups of fresh vegetables along with protein from the egg. The flavorful spices and cheese pull it all together to deliver a savory dish that's bound to become a family favorite.

SERVES: *4*

PREP TIME: *5 minutes*

COOK TIME: *15 minutes*

1 tablespoon olive oil

2 garlic cloves, crushed, or 2 teaspoons jarred, minced garlic

½ cup diced yellow onion

2 teaspoons paprika

1 teaspoon ground cumin

1 teaspoon red pepper flakes (optional)

1 (28-ounce) can crushed tomatoes, no-salt-added

6 ounces fresh spinach, chopped

4 large eggs

¼ cup (1-ounce) feta cheese, crumbled and divided

1. In a soup pot, heat the oil over medium heat.

2. Add the garlic and onion, and sauté for about 3 minutes.

3. Add the paprika, cumin, red pepper flakes (if using), and tomatoes with their juice. Simmer for 5 minutes.

4. Add the spinach and stir for about 1 minute, or until wilted.

5. Carefully crack each egg into the tomato and spinach mixture so they stay separated.

6. Cover and simmer for 3 to 5 minutes, or until the egg yolk is at the desired consistency.

7. Divide into 4 servings and top each with 1 tablespoon of feta cheese.

SUBSTITUTE! *If you don't have fresh spinach on hand, use 10 ounces frozen spinach instead. Make sure to increase the cooking time by 5 minutes.*

STORAGE: *If you make the stew in advance (without the egg and cheese), it can be stored in the refrigerator for up to five days. When you're ready to eat, cook one egg to your prefer-ence for each serving and serve on top of the reheated stew.*

SHORTCUT! *To cut down on cooking time, use four sliced hard-boiled eggs instead of raw eggs. Divide the stew, then add the hard-boiled eggs to each serving.*

Per serving: Calories: 230, Total Fat: 11g, Protein: 14g, Carbohydrates: 21g, Sugars: 13g, Fiber: 8g, Sodium: 482mg

CARROT APPLE SOUP WITH TURMERIC

VEGETARIAN · VEGAN · GLUTEN-FREE · NUT-FREE · DAIRY-FREE

Turmeric is a root that looks similar to fresh ginger. When it is broken or cut open, it is a bright orange-yellow color similar to carrots. The powdered version is widely available and is what gives this soup its distinctive color. Turmeric has also been shown to fight cancer, support eye and liver health, and even aid in weight loss. Coupled with the carrots (known for similar health benefits) and the filling, high-fiber apple, this soup delivers tons of the antioxidants and nutrition you need on your weight loss journey.

SERVES: *4*

PREP TIME: *10 minutes*

COOK TIME: *30 minutes*

1 tablespoon olive oil

½ cup diced onion

1 cup chopped green apple

2 garlic cloves or 2 teaspoons jarred, minced garlic

2 teaspoons ground turmeric

2 cups diced carrots

4 cups low-sodium vegetable broth

1 teaspoon dried thyme

¼ cup plain, fat-free Greek yogurt (optional)

1. In a soup pot, heat the olive oil over medium heat.

2. Add the onion and apple. Sauté for 6 to 8 minutes.

3. Add the garlic and turmeric. Sauté for 30 seconds.

4. Add the carrots, broth, and thyme. Bring to a boil, reduce the heat to low, and simmer for 20 minutes.

5. Use a masher or immersion blender to mash or purée the vegetables and thicken the soup.

6. Divide into 4 servings and top each with 1 tablespoon of yogurt (if using).

SUBSTITUTE! *If you're in a pinch and don't have ground turmeric on hand, you can use 2 teaspoons of curry powder instead. Curry powder contains turmeric and many other spices and will provide a similar flavor and color to turmeric.*

STORAGE: *Store in the refrigerator for up to four days or in the freezer for up to six months.*

Per serving: Calories: 109, Total Fat: 4g, Protein: 3g, Carbohydrates: 17g, Sugars: 9g, Fiber: 3g, Sodium: 110mg

LENTIL SOUP WITH COLLARD GREENS

VEGETARIAN · VEGAN · GLUTEN-FREE · NUT-FREE · DAIRY-FREE

This soup is low in calories but high in nutritional value. Lentils are a great source of dietary protein and help to sustain energy and support metabolism. Likewise, collard greens contain loads of fiber, phytonutrients, and the various vitamins you need on a daily basis.

SERVES: *4*

PREP TIME: *10 minutes*

COOK TIME: *30 minutes*

1 tablespoon olive oil

1 cup sliced carrots

½ cup diced celery

½ cup diced onions

2 garlic cloves or 2 teaspoons jarred, minced garlic

2 teaspoons minced ginger

4 cups low-sodium vegetable broth

2 cups frozen corn

1 cup lentils, green, brown, or red

1 pound collard greens, chopped

1. In a soup pot, heat the olive oil over medium heat. Add the carrots, celery, and onion. Sauté for 3 to 5 minutes.

2. Add the garlic and ginger. Sauté for 30 seconds.

3. Add the broth, corn, and lentils. Stir, bring to a boil, then reduce the heat to low.

4. Simmer for 14 to 18 minutes if using red lentils and 20 to 24 minutes if using green or brown lentils.

5. Add the collard greens and stir for 2 minutes, or until wilted.

6. Divide into 4 servings.

SUBSTITUTE! *Depending on your nutritional goals and taste preferences, you can use any mix of fresh greens such as kale, spinach, or Swiss chard in place of the collard greens.*

STORAGE: *Store in the refrigerator for up to one week or in the freezer for up to two months.*

SHORTCUT! *Save time by using the prechopped bagged greens instead of chopping fresh collard greens.*

Per serving: Calories: 336, Total Fat: 6g, Protein: 20g, Carbohydrates: 56g, Sugars: 6g, Fiber: 22g, Sodium: 133mg

TORTELLINI SOUP WITH CHICKPEAS

VEGETARIAN · NUT-FREE · 30 MINUTES OR LESS

This tortellini soup is a great dinner choice during the fall and winter, complete with tomatoes and carrots. Rich in numerous vitamins and minerals, chickpeas also offer plenty of protein and fiber. As a result, they support digestion, weight loss, satiety, heart health, blood sugar control, and more.

SERVES: *4*

PREP TIME: *5 minutes*

COOK TIME: *20 minutes*

4 cups low-sodium vegetable broth

2 cups water

1 (14-ounce) can diced tomatoes, no-salt-added

1 cup diced carrots

2 teaspoons Italian seasoning

1 (15½-ounce) can chickpeas, drained and rinsed

1 (12-ounce) package dried cheese tortellini

1. In a soup pot, heat the broth, water, tomatoes, carrots, and Italian seasoning over medium heat.

2. Bring to a boil and add the chickpeas and tortellini.

3. Return to a boil, then reduce the heat to low.

4. Simmer for 10 minutes, or until the tortellini are cooked through.

5. Divide into 4 servings.

SUBSTITUTE! *If you can't find dried tortellini, use fresh or frozen tortellini instead. All you have to do is adjust the cooking time according to the package directions. If you can't find chickpeas, look for garbanzo beans. They are the same thing, just with a different name depending on the cuisine.*

STORAGE: *Store in the refrigerator for up to five days.*

Per serving: Calories: 416, Total Fat: 8g, Protein: 19g, Carbohydrates: 69g, Sugars: 7g, Fiber: 7g, Sodium: 362mg

PASTA E FAGIOLI

NUT-FREE • DAIRY-FREE

Pasta e fagioli is a traditional Italian soup with pasta, beans, beef, and vegetables. The name of the dish means "pasta and beans" in Italian. The pasta most often used in this soup is ditalini, which means "little thimbles." If you cannot find them, substitute small shells or orzo instead.

SERVES: *6*

PREP TIME: *10 minutes*

COOK TIME: *25 minutes*

1 pound lean ground beef

1 cup diced carrots

½ cup diced onions

½ cup diced celery

1 (14½-ounce) can diced tomatoes, no-salt-added

1 (15-ounce) can tomato sauce, no-salt-added

1 tablespoon Italian seasoning

4 cups low-sodium beef broth

1 (15-ounce) can great Northern beans, drained and rinsed

1 cup ditalini pasta

1. In a soup pot, brown the beef over medium-high heat for about 5 minutes. Drain any fat.

2. Add the carrots, onions, and celery. Cook with the meat for 3 to 5 minutes.

3. Add the diced tomatoes and their juice, tomato sauce, Italian seasoning, broth, and beans. Bring to a boil.

4. Add the pasta and reduce the heat to low. Simmer for 10 minutes, or until the pasta is fully cooked.

5. Divide into 6 servings.

SUBSTITUTE! *If you don't have Great Northern beans on hand, you can use cannellini beans or navy beans instead.*

STORAGE: *Store in the refrigerator for up to four days.*

SHORTCUT! *If you're low on seasonings or want to skip additional measuring, choose diced tomatoes and tomato sauce with basil, garlic, and oregano and skip the Italian seasoning.*

Per serving: Calories: 257, Total Fat: 7g, Protein: 23g, Carbohydrates: 28g, Sugars: 7g, Fiber: 6g, Sodium: 404mg

CHICKEN AND DUMPLINGS

NUT-FREE • DAIRY-FREE • 30 MINUTES OR LESS

This twist on a classic dish cuts down on both cooking and cleanup time—without sacrificing the savory flavor you know and love. Using gnocchi is a great shortcut for faster dumplings without having to mix them in a separate bowl. Gnocchi are small potato dumplings that are in the dried pasta aisle, in the freezer aisle, or with other "fresh" pasta in the refrigerated section of the grocery store. They typically take about 3 to 5 minutes to cook, but double-check the package directions. Once they're combined with the flavorful chicken, broth, and herbs, they are guaranteed to become a favorite dish for the whole family.

SERVES: *4*

PREP TIME: *5 minutes*

COOK TIME: *20 minutes*

4 cups diced, cooked chicken

4 cups low-sodium
  chicken broth

1 (16-ounce) package frozen
  mixed vegetables including
  carrots, corn, green beans,
  and peas

1 teaspoon dried oregano

1 teaspoon dried basil

1 (12-ounce) package
  potato gnocchi

1. In a soup pot, bring the chicken, broth, vegetables, oregano, and basil to a boil over medium-high heat.

2. Add the gnocchi, stirring to ensure that no dumplings are stuck together.

3. Return to a boil, then reduce the heat to low. Simmer for 5 minutes, or until the gnocchi are fully cooked.

4. Divide into 4 servings.

STORAGE: *Store in the refrigerator for up to four days.*

Per serving: Calories: 478, Total Fat: 7g, Protein: 55g, Carbohydrates: 45g, Sugars: 4g, Fiber: 6g, Sodium: 386mg

CHICKEN PESTO SOUP

30 MINUTES OR LESS

The texture of this soup will remind you of chicken and rice soup, but it contains a lot more nutrients from the beans and spinach. The key to achieving this texture is by using pearl or Israeli couscous. This couscous is larger than traditional white couscous and looks like little balls. It is wheat-based and similar to barley in size but cooks faster, making this dish an excellent option for a quick lunch or weeknight dinner.

SERVES: *4*

PREP TIME: *5 minutes*

COOK TIME: *25 minutes*

4 cups low-sodium chicken broth

½ cup pearl or Israeli couscous

2 cups cubed cooked chicken

1 (15½-ounce) can great Northern beans, drained and rinsed

6 ounces fresh spinach, chopped

⅓ cup pesto sauce

¼ cup grated Parmesan cheese

1. In a soup pot, bring the chicken broth to a boil over medium-high heat.

2. Add the couscous and return to a boil. Reduce the heat to low and simmer for 8 to 10 minutes.

3. Add the chicken and beans and cook for 2 to 3 minutes, or until heated through.

4. Remove from the heat. Stir in the fresh spinach, stirring to wilt, and add the pesto.

5. Divide into 4 servings and top each with 1 tablespoon of Parmesan cheese.

SUBSTITUTE! *If your local grocery store doesn't have pearl or Israeli couscous, you can use ½ cup of orzo pasta instead.*

STORAGE: *Store in the refrigerator for up to four days or in the freezer for up to six months.*

Per serving: Calories: 418, Total Fat: 14g, Protein: 37g, Carbohydrates: 35g, Sugars: 2g, Fiber: 7g, Sodium: 353mg

BEEF STEW

GLUTEN-FREE • NUT-FREE • DAIRY-FREE

Some traditional beef stew recipes can take several hours to cook. In this dish, smaller cuts that cook faster are used. This recipe also skips the addition of flour, which creates a thicker sauce. For a thicker broth, cook for an additional 10 to 15 minutes.

SERVES: *6*

PREP TIME: *15 minutes*

COOK TIME: *45 minutes*

2 tablespoons olive oil, divided

1 cup sliced carrots

1 cup quartered small red potatoes

½ cup diced onions

½ cup diced celery

2 garlic cloves, minced, or 2 teaspoons jarred, minced garlic

1 teaspoon paprika

1 teaspoon dried thyme

1 pound beef stew meat, cut into 1-inch pieces

4 cups low-sodium beef broth

1. In a soup pot, heat 1 tablespoon of olive oil over medium heat.

2. Add the carrots, potatoes, onions, celery, garlic, paprika, and thyme. Cook for 3 to 5 minutes.

3. Add the remaining oil, then add the meat and brown for 5 minutes.

4. Add the broth, bring to a simmer, and reduce the heat to low. Simmer for 25 to 30 minutes, or until the vegetables are easily pierced with a fork.

SUBSTITUTE! *Depending on what you have on hand, you can use lean ground beef instead of stew meat.*

STORAGE: *Store in the refrigerator for up to four days or in the freezer for up to six months.*

SHORTCUT! *To save time dicing vegetables, use 16 ounces of frozen stew vegetables (potatoes, carrots, onions, and celery) in place of the fresh vegetables.*

Per serving: Calories: 183, Total Fat: 9g, Protein: 17g, Carbohydrates: 6g, Sugars: 2g, Fiber: 1g, Sodium: 61mg

CHOCOLATE OAT NUT DESSERT DROPS

VEGETARIAN • GLUTEN-FREE • 30 MINUTES OR LESS

This is a rich dessert that is divided into small portions. The banana makes it naturally sweet, so using dark chocolate (65-percent to 72-percent cocoa) will keep it from becoming too sweet. When shopping, remember that the riper the banana, the more naturally occurring sugars it will have.

SERVES: *16*

PREP TIME: *5 minutes*

COOK TIME: *10 minutes*

1 cup old-fashioned rolled oats

1 cup nonfat milk

1 ripe banana, mashed

2 tablespoons cocoa powder

2 ounces bittersweet or 72% dark chocolate, cut or broken into pieces

½ cup chopped pecans

1 teaspoon vanilla extract

1. In a saucepan or small soup pot, combine the oats, milk, banana, and cocoa powder. Cook over medium-low heat, stirring constantly to prevent the milk from burning, for about 5 minutes.

2. Remove from the heat and add the chocolate pieces, stirring to melt.

3. Stir in the pecans and vanilla.

4. Using a tablespoon, drop 16 individual servings onto a plate or baking sheet lined with parchment paper. Put in the refrigerator or freezer until firm.

5. When firm, store in an airtight container in the freezer or refrigerator. They can also be kept at room temperature.

STORAGE: *Store in the refrigerator for up to one month or in the freezer for up to six months. If storing at room temperature, it will keep for up to two weeks.*

Per serving: Calories: 80, Total Fat: 5g, Protein: 2g, Carbohydrates: 8g, Sugars: 3g, Fiber: 2g, Sodium: 9mg

CHAPTER 7: NOTES

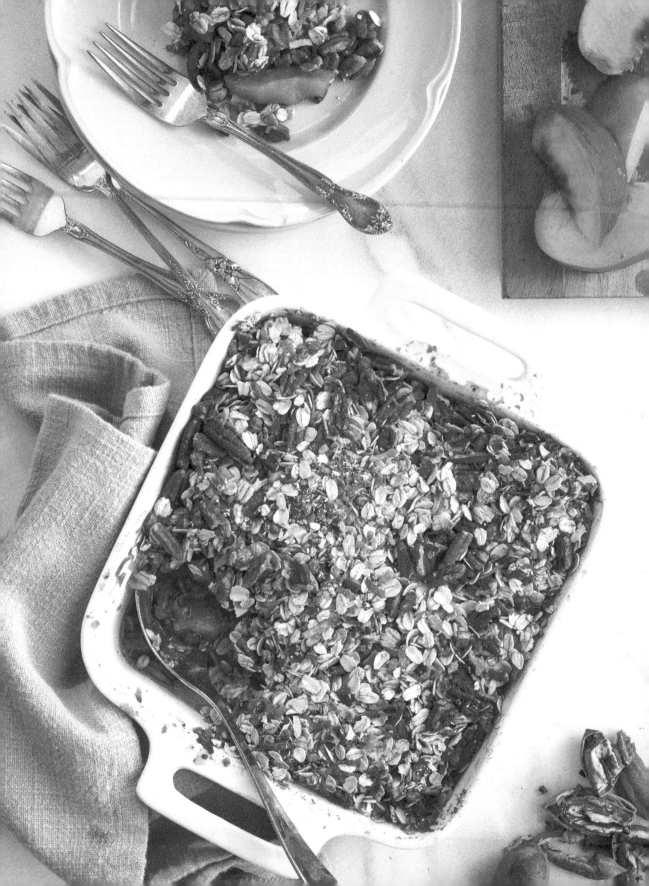

DUTCH OVEN

Dutch ovens are probably one of the most versatile versions of the cooking pot. It doesn't need electricity and can go on both a stovetop and in an oven. They're even used over an open fire when camping. Most of these recipes use the Dutch oven on the stovetop, but for the Peaches with Streusel Topping, you'll be putting it in the oven. Make sure that your Dutch oven has a tight-fitting lid for recipe steps that require simmering.

Because of the larger capacity of this cooking vessel, many of the recipes make large batches. They are great options for make-ahead meals to have on hand throughout the week.

Peaches with
Streusel Topping,
p. 136

BLACK BEAN AND EGG "BURRITO" BOWL

VEGETARIAN · GLUTEN-FREE · NUT-FREE · 30 MINUTES OR LESS

From the black beans to the eggs to the cheese, this burrito-inspired bowl is full of metabolism-supporting protein and tons of flavor. The black beans and green chilies are also packed with plenty of fiber to help you feel full longer and also support digestion. So even if you leave out the optional whole wheat tortillas, this dish will keep you satisfied until lunch.

SERVES: *6*

PREP TIME: *10 minutes*

COOK TIME: *20 minutes*

½ tablespoon olive oil

½ cup diced onions

2 garlic cloves, crushed, or 2 teaspoons jarred, minced garlic

1 (15½-ounce) can black beans, drained and rinsed

1 (10-ounce) can diced tomatoes with green chiles

2 teaspoons chili powder

1 teaspoon ground cumin

1 teaspoon ground coriander

6 large eggs

⅓ cup queso fresco or shredded Mexican blend cheese, divided

6 (8-inch) whole wheat tortillas (optional)

1. In a Dutch oven, heat the oil over medium heat.

2. Add the onion and garlic. Sauté for 3 minutes.

3. Add the black beans, tomatoes with their juice, chili powder, cumin, and coriander. Simmer for 5 minutes.

4. Using a spoon or a ladle, make 6 wells in the bean-tomato mixture.

5. Drop one egg in each well. Cover and cook for 7 to 10 minutes, or until the egg yolk is cooked to your preference.

6. Divide into 6 servings and top each with 1 tablespoon of cheese.

7. Serve in or with the tortillas (if using).

SUBSTITUTE! *If you prefer a less spicy dish, you can use 1 (14¼-ounce) can of diced tomatoes instead of the diced tomatoes with green chilies.*

SHORTCUT! *To save some time, make the bean-tomato mixture as directed, divide into 6 servings, and serve with hard-boiled eggs instead of cooking the eggs in the Dutch oven.*

Per serving: Calories: 371, Total Fat: 16g, Protein: 17g, Carbohydrates: 42g, Sugars: 4g, Fiber: 9g, Sodium: 466mg

SAVORY OATMEAL
WITH TOMATOES AND AVOCADOS

VEGETARIAN · VEGAN · GLUTEN-FREE · NUT-FREE · 30 MINUTES OR LESS

Most people think of oatmeal as a sweet breakfast dish, but once you go the savory route with this recipe—packed with vegetables, seeds, and flavorful vinegar—you won't miss the sweeter versions. There are many options, so experiment with what you prefer, keeping the ratios the same.

SERVES: *6*

PREP TIME: *5 minutes*

COOK TIME: *10 minutes*

6 cups water

3 cups old-fashioned rolled oats

12 ounces (about 20) grape tomatoes, halved

3 tablespoons balsamic vinegar

¼ cup grated Parmesan cheese

3 tablespoons sunflower seeds

2 medium avocados, sliced in thirds

1. In a Dutch oven, bring the water to a boil. Add the oats and reduce the heat to low and simmer. Cook the oats for 5 minutes, stirring occasionally.

2. Remove from the heat and stir in the tomatoes, balsamic vinegar, and cheese.

3. Divide into 6 servings and top each with ½ tablespoon of sunflower seeds and one-third of the avocado slices.

SUBSTITUTE! *Pumpkin seeds have been associated with reduced risk of bladder conditions and may be used in place of sunflower seeds if you're looking to support urinary health.*

STORAGE: *Store in the refrigerator for up to three days.*

Per serving: Calories: 288, Total Fat: 14g, Protein: 9g, Carbohydrates: 36g, Sugars: 2g, Fiber: 9g, Sodium: 53mg

SWEET POTATO KALE SOUP

VEGETARIAN · VEGAN · GLUTEN-FREE · NUT-FREE · DAIRY-FREE

Sweet potatoes and yams are terms often used interchangeably, but they are not the same thing. Yams have a lighter-color flesh and are much starchier and less sweet than sweet potatoes. Sweet potatoes can have white, pale yellow, orange, or even purple flesh and are a good source of the vitamin A precursor, beta-carotene. Despite the name, sweet potatoes are often used in savory dishes like this one. In this recipe, the sweet potato balances out more bitter vegetables, such as kale.

SERVES: *6*

PREP TIME: *10 minutes*

COOK TIME: *30 minutes*

1 tablespoon olive oil

1 cup diced onion

3 garlic cloves, crushed, or 1 tablespoon jarred, minced garlic

1½ pounds sweet potatoes, peeled and diced

1 (14½-ounce) can diced tomatoes, no-salt-added

1 (6-ounce) can tomato paste, no-salt-added

2 (15½-ounce) cans great Northern beans

5 cups water

1 teaspoon ground cumin

1 teaspoon salt

½ teaspoon freshly ground black pepper

1 pound kale, chopped

1. In a Dutch oven, heat the oil over medium heat.

2. Add the onion and garlic. Sauté for 3 minutes.

3. Add the sweet potatoes, tomatoes with their juice, tomato paste, beans, water, cumin, salt, and pepper. Bring to boil.

4. Reduce the heat to low and bring to a simmer. Cover and cook for 20 minutes.

5. Remove from the heat and then add the kale, stirring to wilt.

6. Divide into 6 servings.

SUBSTITUTE! *If you don't have Great Northern beans on hand, you can use one (15 ½-ounce) can of chickpeas instead.*

STORAGE: *Store in the refrigerator for up to five days or freeze for up to six months.*

SHORTCUT! *To save some time, you can use two (10-ounce) bags of frozen diced sweet potatoes instead of fresh sweet potatoes.*

Per serving: Calories: 301, Total Fat: 4g, Protein: 11g, Carbohydrates: 59g, Sugars: 12g, Fiber: 14g, Sodium: 457mg

SHRIMP WITH VEGETABLES AND HONEY SOY SAUCE

NUT-FREE • DAIRY-FREE

When purchasing shrimp, you can expect to get 30 to 40 medium shrimp per pound. To save time and mess, buy them peeled. Most come with their tails still on, even when peeled. When buying fresh shrimp, use them within a day, or keep frozen shrimp on hand so that it's readily available for this recipe. If you use frozen shrimp, defrost them in the refrigerator for 24 hours before using them here. The mix of honey and soy sauce in this recipe balances out the salty and sweet flavors just right.

SERVES: *4*

PREP TIME: *15 minutes*

COOK TIME: *10 minutes*

1 tablespoon olive oil

½ cup diced celery

1 cup sliced carrots

½ cup snap peas, trimmed

1 garlic clove, crushed, or 1 teaspoon jarred, minced garlic

½ teaspoon minced ginger

1 pound medium raw shrimp, peeled and tails removed

3 tablespoons honey

2 tablespoons low-sodium soy sauce

1. In a Dutch oven, heat the oil over medium heat for 1 minute.

2. Add the celery, carrots, snap peas, and garlic. Sauté for 5 minutes, or until the vegetables are tender.

3. Add the ginger and sauté for 30 seconds.

4. Add the shrimp, stir, and cook for 2 to 4 minutes, or until cooked through. Remove from the heat.

5. Add the honey and soy sauce, stirring to mix.

6. Divide into 4 servings.

SUBSTITUTE! *For a different flavor profile and to take advantage of the vitamin C and antioxidants in bell peppers, substitute red, yellow, or orange bell peppers in place of the carrots.*

SHORTCUT! *For easier cleanup and measuring, use the same tablespoon to measure the oil, honey, and soy sauce. Using the same measuring spoon first for the oil and then for the honey will help the honey pour off the spoon easily.*

Per serving: Calories: 223, Total Fat: 5g, Protein: 26g, Carbohydrates: 20g, Sugars: 16g, Fiber: 2g, Sodium: 625mg

CHICKEN BUTTERNUT SQUASH PEANUT STEW

GLUTEN-FREE • DAIRY-FREE

Using peanut butter in stew may sound unusual, but it is a classic West African flavor profile. Here it combines with chicken and squash for a hearty, savory meal. Peanut butter has a natural balance of healthy fats and plant-based protein, which will support satiety and prevent you from feeling hungry just a few hours later. Don't choose reduced-fat peanut butter—in which healthy fat is removed and more sugar is added. If possible, go for the all-natural option.

SERVES: *8*

PREP TIME: *10 minutes*

COOK TIME: *30 minutes*

2 tablespoons olive oil

1½ pounds boneless, skinless chicken, cut into 1-inch pieces

1 cup diced onions

1 tablespoon minced ginger or ½ teaspoon ground ginger

2 garlic cloves, crushed, or 2 teaspoons jarred, minced garlic

2 (10-ounce) packages frozen butternut squash

1 (14½-ounce) can crushed tomatoes, no-salt-added

4 cups low-sodium chicken broth

1 to 2 tablespoons red pepper flakes

½ cup creamy peanut butter

1. In a Dutch oven, heat the oil over medium heat.

2. Add the chicken, onion, ginger, and garlic. Sauté for 5 minutes.

3. Add the butternut squash, crushed tomatoes with their juice, broth, and red pepper flakes. Bring to a boil.

4. Stir in the peanut butter. Reduce the heat to low and simmer, covered, for 20 minutes.

5. Divide into 8 servings.

SUBSTITUTE! *While butternut squash has fewer calories, you can use 20 ounces of frozen diced sweet potato instead to increase the amount of fiber and protein in this dish.*

STORAGE: *Store in the refrigerator for up to four days or in the freezer for up to six months.*

Per serving: Calories: 290, Total Fat: 14g, Protein: 25g, Carbohydrates: 19g, Sugars: 7g, Fiber: 5g, Sodium: 259mg

LEMON CHICKEN THIGHS WITH ARTICHOKE HEARTS

GLUTEN-FREE · NUT-FREE · DAIRY-FREE · 30 MINUTES OR LESS

Artichokes are often overlooked as an ingredient in cooking because they are considered too labor-intensive to prepare. By using jarred or canned artichoke hearts, you save the time of trimming and cooking them, and they are low in calories, too, with only 90 calories in the entire 14-ounce jar. Their mild flavor pairs well with the chicken and lemon to create a delicious dinner.

SERVES: *4*

PREP TIME: *15 minutes*

COOK TIME: *25 minutes*

1 tablespoon olive oil

1 pound boneless, skinless chicken thighs

½ teaspoon salt, divided

½ teaspoon freshly ground black pepper, divided

1 (14-ounce) can quartered artichoke hearts, drained and rinsed

1 cup low-sodium chicken broth

2 lemons, sliced thin and seeded

2 cups hot, cooked brown rice

1. In a Dutch oven, heat the oil over medium heat.

2. Add the chicken thighs, ¼ teaspoon of the salt, and ¼ teaspoon of the pepper. Brown for about 3 minutes, then flip the chicken and add the remaining ¼ teaspoon of salt and ¼ teaspoon of pepper. Brown for 3 minutes.

3. Add the artichokes and broth. Bring to a simmer and cook for 10 minutes.

4. Add the lemons and simmer for another 2 minutes.

5. Divide the rice into 4 servings and top each with the chicken mixture and sauce.

STORAGE: *Store in the refrigerator for up to four days.*

SHORTCUT! *To save some prep time and cut down on cleanup, use precooked brown rice, which can be found in the freezer or grain aisle in your grocery store.*

Per serving: Calories: 282, Total Fat: 9g, Protein: 26g, Carbohydrates: 25g, Sugars: 2g, Fiber: 5g, Sodium: 630mg

PORK LOIN WITH APPLES AND ONIONS

GLUTEN-FREE • NUT-FREE • DAIRY-FREE

"Loin" is a leaner cut of meat. If there is visible fat on the edges of the pork chop, make sure to trim it before cooking. The combination of the apples and onions make for a unique sweet and savory flavor that goes well with pork.

SERVES: *4*

PREP TIME: *10 minutes*

COOK TIME: *20 minutes*

2 tablespoons olive oil

1 tablespoon Dijon mustard

1 teaspoon dried rosemary or 1 tablespoon chopped fresh rosemary

1 teaspoon salt

½ teaspoon freshly ground black pepper

1 pound boneless pork loin chops, cut into 4 pieces

1 cup low-sodium chicken broth

2 Granny Smith apples, cored and sliced

2 medium red onions (the same size as the apples), quartered

1. In a Dutch oven, heat the olive oil over medium heat.

2. Spread the mustard, rosemary, salt, and pepper evenly over both sides of the pork chops.

3. Add the pork chops to the pan and brown for 2 to 3 minutes on each side.

4. Add the broth and scrape the bottom of the Dutch oven to remove any browned pieces. Simmer for 1 minute.

5. Add the apples and onions. Cover and cook for 10 to 12 minutes, until the apples and onions are tender and the pork is cooked through.

6. Divide into 4 servings.

STORAGE: *Store in the refrigerator for up to four days.*

Per serving: Calories: 367, Total Fat: 20g, Protein: 27g, Carbohydrates: 22g, Sugars: 14g, Fiber: 4g, Sodium: 987mg

PIZZA CASSEROLE

NUT-FREE

This recipe provides the best of both worlds: the taste mimics a pizza with toppings such as ground beef, onions, mushrooms, and peppers, but without the calories you'd get from placing an order at your favorite pizzeria. For a low-calorie twist, you can add black olives to the final dish if you like them on your slice.

SERVES: *6*

PREP TIME: *10 minutes*

COOK TIME: *30 minutes*

1 pound lean ground beef

½ cup diced onions

4 ounces white mushrooms, sliced

1 medium red bell pepper, sliced

1 (24-ounce) jar pizza sauce

2 cups water

2 teaspoons dried oregano

2 teaspoons dried basil

8 ounces (about 3 cups) whole wheat rotini pasta

¾ cup shredded mozzarella cheese, divided

1. In a Dutch oven, brown the ground beef over medium heat for 4 to 5 minutes. Drain the fat.

2. Add the onions, mushrooms, and bell pepper. Sauté for 3 minutes.

3. Add the pizza sauce, water, oregano, and basil. Bring to a boil, reduce the heat to low, and simmer.

4. Add the pasta. Cover and cook for 10 to 12 minutes, or until the pasta is cooked.

5. Divide into 6 servings and top each with 2 tablespoons of cheese.

SUBSTITUTE! *Depending on what you have on hand, you can use 1 (24-ounce) jar of low-sugar or no-sugar-added marinara sauce in place of the pizza sauce.*

Per serving: Calories: 309, Total Fat: 10g, Protein: 47g, Carbohydrates: 32g, Sugars: 6g, Fiber: 5g, Sodium: 582mg

STOVETOP LASAGNA WITH SHREDDED CARROTS

NUT-FREE

While this dish doesn't have the "stacked" look of traditional lasagna, it does have all the components, along with the added benefit of shredded vegetables in the tomato and meat mix. Between the lasagna noodles and the carrots, you'll feel full and satisfied after eating a serving of this hearty meal. It also reheats well for lunch the following day.

SERVES: 6

PREP TIME: *10 minutes*

COOK TIME: *20 minutes*

1 pound lean ground beef

½ cup diced onions

1 cup shredded carrots

1 (24-ounce) jar marinara sauce, no-sugar-added

1 cup water

1 tablespoon Italian seasoning

8 ounces oven-ready lasagna noodles

1 cup low-fat ricotta cheese

¾ cup shredded mozzarella cheese, divided

1. In a Dutch oven, brown the ground beef and onions over medium heat for 4 to 5 minutes. Drain the fat.

2. Add the carrots, marinara sauce, water, and Italian seasoning. Bring to a boil, then reduce the heat to low and simmer.

3. Break up the lasagna noodles into 2-inch pieces and stir them into the sauce.

4. Spread the ricotta cheese on top of the sauce and stir once to mix it in slightly.

5. Cover and continue to simmer for 10 to 12 minutes.

6. Divide into 6 servings and top each with 2 tablespoons of mozzarella cheese.

SUBSTITUTE! *While ricotta contains fewer calories, you can use 1 cup of cottage cheese instead, depending on what you have on hand.*

STORAGE: *Store in the refrigerator for up to four days.*

Per serving: Calories: 422, Total Fat: 13g, Protein: 30g, Carbohydrates: 45g, Sugars: 11g, Fiber: 4g, Sodium: 255mg

PEACHES WITH STREUSEL TOPPING

VEGETARIAN · VEGAN · GLUTEN-FREE · DAIRY-FREE · 30 MINUTES OR LESS

Stone fruits have flesh that surrounds a stone-like pit. They include apricots, cherries, mangoes, nectarine, peaches, and plums. In fact, nectarines and peaches are related. Interestingly, nectarines are a type of peach, but not all peaches are nectarines. Here, you can use either fruit since their nutrition profiles are the same, but any mix of stone fruit would make this a delicious dessert.

SERVES: *8*

PREP TIME: *10 minutes*

COOK TIME: *15 minutes*

8 to 10 (about 2½ pounds) peaches or nectarines, sliced and stones removed

⅓ cup pure maple syrup

1 cup old-fashioned oats

1 cup chopped pecans

½ cup shredded coconut

2 teaspoons ground cinnamon

1. Preheat the oven to 350°F.

2. In a Dutch oven, toss the peaches with maple syrup to coat.

3. Sprinkle the oats, pecans, coconut, and cinnamon over the peaches.

4. Bake for 15 minutes, or until the peaches are heated through.

5. Divide into 8 servings and serve warm.

SUBSTITUTE! *If you don't have fresh peaches on hand, you can use frozen sliced peaches instead. Just increase the baking time to 25 minutes. You can also use apricots, plums, or any mix of stone fruits for variety.*

STORAGE: *Store in the refrigerator for up to one week.*

Per serving: Calories: 212, Total Fat: 12g, Protein: 3g, Carbohydrates: 23g, Sugars: 13g, Fiber: 4g, Sodium: 3mg

CHAPTER 8: NOTES

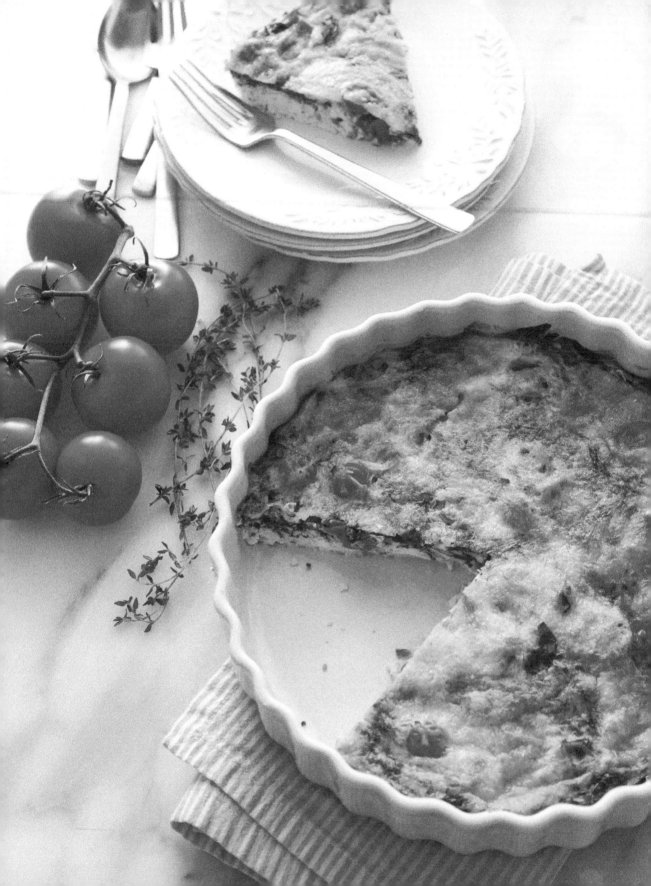

CASSEROLE DISH AND SHEET PAN

This chapter contains recipes made exclusively in the oven using either a baking sheet, casserole dish, or baking pan.

In most of them, the baking sheet size is 9-by-13 inches. Using parchment paper or aluminum foil to line the baking sheet makes cleanup easier and prevents food from sticking.

A baking pan is often made of glass and is either 9-by-13 inches or 9-by-9 inches. Other casserole dishes will work, but they may affect cooking times.

Crustless Breakfast
Quiche, p. 142

BREAKFASTS

BAKED OATMEAL WITH BLUEBERRIES 141

CRUSTLESS BREAKFAST QUICHE 142

MAIN DISHES

SALMON WITH BROCCOLI AND ZUCCHINI 143

BAKED TILAPIA WITH TOMATOES
AND GREEN BEANS 144

CHICKEN AND BEAN ENCHILADA
CASSEROLE 145

CHICKEN AND RICE WITH BROCCOLI
AND SQUASH 146

GARLIC CHICKEN WITH ASPARAGUS
AND MUSHROOMS 147

PORK TENDERLOIN WITH ROOT VEGETABLES
AND ORANGE HONEY SAUCE 148

BEEF WITH POTATOES AND BROCCOLI 149

DESSERT

MIXED BERRY CRISP 150

BAKED OATMEAL WITH BLUEBERRIES

VEGETARIAN · GLUTEN-FREE · NUT-FREE

This baked oatmeal can be served the morning it is prepared or made ahead for a grab-and-go meal during hectic weekdays. The combination of cinnamon, maple syrup, and vanilla give this dish a flavor the whole family will love. Of all fruits and vegetables, blueberries contain some of the highest levels of antioxidants, which are known to fight the free radicals that can contribute to many diseases.

SERVES: *8*

PREP TIME: *5 minutes*

COOK TIME: *30 minutes*

Nonstick cooking spray

3 cups old-fashioned rolled oats

2 teaspoons ground cinnamon

2 teaspoons baking powder

½ cup pure maple syrup

1 cup nonfat milk

3 large eggs

2 teaspoons vanilla extract

2 cups blueberries, fresh or frozen

1. Preheat the oven to 350°F. Spray a 9-by-13-inch glass or metal pan with cooking spray.

2. Spread the oats, cinnamon, and baking powder in the pan.

3. Pour the maple syrup evenly over the oats.

4. In a 2-cup measuring cup, stir the milk, eggs, and vanilla with a fork until well combined. Pour evenly over the oat mixture.

5. Spread the blueberries evenly on top.

6. Bake for 30 minutes, or until set.

7. Cut into 8 pieces and serve.

SUBSTITUTE! *Depending on what you have on hand, you can use sliced bananas or strawberries in place of the blueberries.*

STORAGE: *Store individual servings in airtight containers in the refrigerator for up to one week.*

SHORTCUT! *For easier mixing, you can use ¾ cup of liquid eggs instead of the large eggs.*

Per serving: Calories: 233, Total Fat: 4g, Protein: 8g, Carbohydrates: 42g, Sugars: 17g, Fiber: 4g, Sodium: 47mg

CRUSTLESS BREAKFAST QUICHE

VEGETARIAN • GLUTEN-FREE • NUT-FREE

Quiche traditionally has a crust made from fat, flour, and water. Eliminating the crust cuts a large portion of the less-healthy calories. It's used to prevent sticking, so without it, be sure that the casserole pan is sprayed with cooking spray to keep the eggs from sticking. This dish can be made on prep day and served throughout the week.

SERVES: *8*

PREP TIME: *10 minutes*

COOK TIME: *40 minutes*

Nonstick cooking spray

8 large eggs

1¼ cup nonfat milk

1 teaspoon dried thyme

1 teaspoon salt

½ teaspoon freshly ground
  black pepper

2 cups chopped
  baby spinach

1 cup halved grape or
  cherry tomatoes

1 cup shredded Swiss cheese

1. Preheat the oven to 375°F. Spray a 9-by-13-inch glass pan with a generous amount of cooking spray.

2. In a 4-cup liquid measuring cup, stir the eggs and milk with a fork until well combined. Pour into the prepared dish.

3. Sprinkle the thyme, salt, and pepper evenly over the egg and milk mixture.

4. Add the spinach and tomatoes, spreading evenly. Using a fork, press the vegetables into the egg mixture.

5. Sprinkle the cheese evenly on top.

6. Bake for 40 minutes, or until cooked through.

7. Divide into 8 servings.

SUBSTITUTE! *Depending on your nutritional and health goals, you can use 3 cups of vegetables in any combination in place of the spinach and tomatoes, such as chopped broccoli florets, asparagus, and sliced mushrooms.*

STORAGE: *Store in the refrigerator for up to four days.*

SHORTCUT! *For easier blending, you can use 2 cups liquid eggs in place of the large eggs.*

Per serving: Calories: 143, Total Fat: 9g, Protein: 12g, Carbohydrates: 4g, Sugars: 3g, Fiber: 1g, Sodium: 414mg

SALMON WITH BROCCOLI AND ZUCCHINI

GLUTEN-FREE • NUT-FREE • DAIRY-FREE • 30 MINUTES OR LESS

Baking salmon is a good way for beginners to learn how to cook fish. The varying thickness of salmon fillets will determine how long the fish needs to be cooked, but if you're using a thermometer, the internal temperature of the fish should be 145°F. This dish will take out a lot of the guesswork and leave you with a savory treat bound to get rave reviews.

SERVES: *4*

PREP TIME: *10 minutes*

COOK TIME: *20 minutes*

3 cups broccoli florets

2 cups sliced zucchini

1 medium red bell
  pepper, sliced

2 tablespoons olive oil

4 (6-ounce) salmon fillets

2 teaspoons dill

1 teaspoon salt

½ teaspoon garlic powder

½ teaspoon freshly ground
  black pepper

1. Preheat the oven to 400°F. Line a 9-by-13-inch sheet pan with parchment paper or aluminum foil.

2. Spread the broccoli, zucchini, and bell pepper evenly on the sheet pan and pour the oil over the top. Bake for 10 minutes.

3. Remove the sheet pan from the oven. Using tongs or a fork, move the vegetables to the side of the pan.

4. Put the salmon skin-side down on the sheet pan and sprinkle with the dill. Sprinkle the salt, garlic powder, and pepper evenly over the vegetables and salmon.

5. Return the pan to the oven and bake for 5 to 8 minutes, or until the salmon is cooked through.

6. Divide into 4 servings.

SUBSTITUTE! *Depending on your taste preferences and what's in season, you can substitute asparagus for the broccoli or a yellow squash for the zucchini.*

STORAGE: *Store in the refrigerator for up to three days.*

Per serving: Calories: 404, Total Fat: 25g, Protein: 36g, Carbohydrates: 9g, Sugars: 4g, Fiber: 3g, Sodium: 509mg

BAKED TILAPIA WITH TOMATOES AND GREEN BEANS

GLUTEN-FREE • NUT-FREE • DAIRY-FREE • 30 MINUTES OR LESS

Tilapia is a white fish that contains mostly protein and is low in fat, with about 25 grams of protein and only 130 calories in a $3\frac{1}{2}$-ounce serving. Other white fish with a similar texture and nutrition are cod, haddock, and bass. Combining this protein-rich fish with tomatoes and green beans provides a well-rounded, balanced meal.

SERVES: *4*

PREP TIME: *5 minutes*

COOK TIME: *20 minutes*

1 pint grape or
   cherry tomatoes

12 ounces fresh green
   beans, trimmed

1 tablespoon olive oil

1 teaspoon salt

½ teaspoon freshly ground
   black pepper

4 (6-ounce) tilapia fillets

2 tablespoons Dijon
   mustard, divided

1 teaspoon tarragon

1 tablespoon lemon juice

1. Preheat the oven to 450°F. Line a 9-by-13-inch sheet pan with parchment paper or foil.

2. Spread the tomatoes and green beans on the sheet pan and drizzle the oil over it, using your hands to evenly coat the vegetables. Sprinkle with the salt and pepper.

3. Move the vegetables to the side of the pan and put the tilapia fillets in the pan.

4. Spread ½ tablespoon of the mustard on each fillet with a knife.

5. Sprinkle the tarragon and lemon juice over the fillets. Bake for 17 to 20 minutes.

6. Remove from the oven and divide into 4 servings.

SUBSTITUTE! *Depending on what you have on hand, you can use four halved Roma tomatoes in place of the cherry or grape tomatoes.*

STORAGE: *Store in the refrigerator for up to three days.*

Per serving: Calories: 234, Total Fat: 6g, Protein: 34g, Carbohydrates: 15g, Sugars: 9g, Fiber: 5g, Sodium: 537mg

CHICKEN AND BEAN ENCHILADA CASSEROLE

GLUTEN-FREE · NUT-FREE

This recipe calls for salsa verde, or green salsa, which is made with onion, garlic, cilantro, hot peppers, and tomatillos. Enchiladas are often rolled up with the ingredients in the tortilla and placed seam-side down in the pan to cook. By stacking the tortillas as in this recipe, however, you're shortening the preparation time.

SERVES: 6

PREP TIME: *10 minutes*

COOK TIME: *35 minutes*

Nonstick cooking spray

1 (24-ounce) jar salsa verde, divided

12 (6-inch) corn tortillas

2 cups shredded cooked chicken, divided

1 (15½-ounce) can pinto beans, drained, rinsed, and divided

1 (20-ounce) package frozen pepper and onion blend

1 teaspoon ground cumin, divided

1 teaspoon garlic powder, divided

1½ cups shredded Monterey Jack cheese, divided

1. Preheat the oven to 375°F. Spray a 9-by-9-inch glass pan or casserole dish with cooking spray.

2. In the bottom of the glass dish, pour ½ cup of salsa verde and spread evenly. Layer four corn tortillas over the salsa verde so they overlap.

3. Layer 1 cup of chicken, ½ can of the pinto beans, and about half the pepper and onion blend over the tortillas.

4. Season the vegetables with ½ teaspoon cumin and ½ teaspoon garlic powder.

5. Pour ¾ cup salsa verde over the vegetables. Top with ½ cup of Monterey Jack cheese.

6. Repeat with a layer of four tortillas and the remaining chicken, pinto beans, pepper and onion blend, cumin, and garlic powder.

7. Top with ¾ cup of salsa verde and ½ cup of Monterey Jack cheese.

8. Add the final four tortillas on top. Put the remaining salsa verde and Monterey Jack cheese over the top.

9. Bake for 35 minutes, or until heated through and the cheese is melted.

10. Divide into 6 servings.

SUBSTITUTE! You can use 1 (15½-ounce) can black beans, drained and rinsed, in place of the pinto beans.

Per serving: Calories: 346, Total Fat: 12g, Protein: 26g, Carbohydrates: 34g, Sugars: 6g, Fiber: 5g, Sodium: 665mg

CHICKEN AND RICE WITH BROCCOLI AND SQUASH

GLUTEN-FREE • NUT-FREE • DAIRY-FREE

Quick-cooking or "minute" rice is rice that has been previously cooked and dehydrated. Using quick-cooking brown rice in this dish ensures that the rice is fully cooked without needing an hour and a separate pot to do so. Make sure to use brown, not white, rice in this dish for an extra boost of nutrients and fiber.

SERVES: *4*

PREP TIME: *5 minutes*

COOK TIME: *40 minutes*

Nonstick cooking spray

1 cup quick-cooking brown rice

1 pound boneless, skinless chicken breast, cut into 1-inch pieces

1 (10-ounce) package frozen diced butternut squash

2 cups broccoli florets

2 teaspoons dried thyme

3 cups low-sodium chicken broth

1. Preheat the oven to 400°F. Spray a 9-by-13-inch glass baking dish with cooking spray.

2. Add the rice, chicken, butternut squash, and broccoli to the baking dish, spreading the ingredients out in an even layer. Season with the thyme.

3. Pour the chicken broth over the chicken mixture in the baking pan.

4. Cover tightly with foil and bake for 30 minutes.

5. Remove the foil and bake for another 10 minutes.

6. Divide into 4 servings.

SUBSTITUTE! *If you're looking to shave off a few calories, you can use cauliflower in place of the broccoli.*

STORAGE: *Store in the refrigerator for up to four days or in the freezer for up to four months.*

SHORTCUT! *To cut down on prep time, you can use 1 (10-ounce) package frozen broccoli florets in place of the fresh broccoli.*

Per serving: Calories: 226, Total Fat: 3g, Protein: 28g, Carbohydrates: 20g, Sugars: 2g, Fiber: 3g, Sodium: 128mg

GARLIC CHICKEN WITH ASPARAGUS AND MUSHROOMS

GLUTEN-FREE • NUT-FREE DAIRY-FREE

Garlic is a major flavor in this dish, but it makes space for the asparagus to get its flavor share in, too. Cooking with garlic has potential benefits to blood pressure, cholesterol levels, and immune function. Meanwhile, the asparagus in this dish contains fiber, folate, and many essential vitamins.

SERVES: *4*

PREP TIME: *10 minutes*

COOK TIME: *25 minutes*

1 pound boneless, skinless chicken breast

6 garlic cloves, crushed, or 2 tablespoons jarred, minced garlic

8 ounces white or baby bella mushrooms, sliced

1 pound asparagus, trimmed

2 tablespoons olive oil

1 teaspoon salt

1 teaspoon lemon pepper

1. Preheat the oven to 400°F. Line a 9-by-13-inch baking sheet with parchment paper or foil.

2. Place the chicken on the baking sheet and spread the garlic on top.

3. Spread the mushrooms and asparagus in an even layer around the chicken.

4. Drizzle the oil evenly over the chicken and vegetables. Season with the salt and pepper.

5. Cook for 22 to 26 minutes, or until the chicken is cooked through.

6. Divide into 4 servings.

STORAGE: *Store in the refrigerator for up to four days.*

SHORTCUT! *If you don't have fresh asparagus on hand or want to plan ahead, you can use frozen asparagus spears instead.*

Per serving: Calories: 225, Total Fat: 9g, Protein: 30g, Carbohydrates: 9g, Sugars: 3g, Fiber: 4g, Sodium: 563mg

PORK TENDERLOIN WITH ROOT VEGETABLES AND ORANGE HONEY SAUCE

GLUTEN-FREE · NUT-FREE · DAIRY-FREE

Root vegetables are vegetables that grow in the ground, such as beets, carrots, onions, sweet potatoes, and turnips. Roasting them makes them caramelize, giving them more flavor. They are great sources of complex carbohydrates and fiber, and they've also been associated with a reduced risk of diabetes.

SERVES: *6*

PREP TIME: *10 minutes*

COOK TIME: *25 minutes*

12 ounces (about 3 medium) sweet potatoes, diced

6 ounces (about 3 medium) carrots, sliced

6 ounces (about 2 small) beets, peeled, diced

2 tablespoons olive oil, divided

1½ pounds pork tenderloin

2 teaspoons dried rosemary

¾ teaspoon salt

¾ teaspoon freshly ground black pepper

Juice of 1 medium orange

1 tablespoon honey

1. Preheat the oven to 400°F. Line a 9-by-13-inch baking sheet with parchment paper or foil.

2. Spread the sweet potatoes, carrots, and beets on the baking sheet in an even layer and drizzle with 1 tablespoon oil.

3. Move the vegetables to the edge of the baking sheet and put the pork in.

4. Drizzle the remaining 1 tablespoon oil evenly over the pork.

5. Season the vegetables and pork with the rosemary, salt, and pepper.

6. Bake for 20 to 25 minutes, or until the pork reaches an internal temperature of 145°F.

7. Pour ¼ cup of orange juice into a liquid measuring cup. Add the honey to the orange juice and stir to combine. Pour this over the pork and vegetables when they come out of the oven.

8. Let the pork rest for 10 minutes, then cut the meat, dividing it evenly into 6 servings.

STORAGE: *Store in the refrigerator for up to four days or freeze individual servings for up to six months.*

Per serving: Calories: 251, Total Fat: 9g, Protein: 22g, Carbohydrates: 22g, Sugars: 10g, Fiber: 3g, Sodium: 428mg

BEEF WITH POTATOES AND BROCCOLI

GLUTEN-FREE • NUT-FREE • DAIRY-FREE

This recipe offers a healthy twist on the traditional "meat and potatoes" meal people love. Rather than making the flank steak the center of the meal, it is about one-third of the meal, which allows for a healthier balance of vegetables and protein. The vegetables in this dish include digestion-supporting onion, broccoli, and bell pepper.

SERVES: *4*

PREP TIME: *10 minutes*

COOK TIME: *20 minutes*

1 medium red onion, cut into 8 pieces

½ pound fingerling potatoes

2 cups broccoli florets

1 cup red bell pepper, diced

1 tablespoon olive oil

1 pound flank steak

1 teaspoon paprika

1 teaspoon ground cumin

1 teaspoon garlic powder

1. Preheat the oven to 400°F. Line a 9-by-13-inch baking sheet with parchment paper or foil.

2. Spread the onion, potatoes, broccoli, and bell pepper on the baking sheet. Drizzle the oil evenly over the vegetables.

3. Move the vegetables aside. Place the steak in the middle of the sheet and spread the vegetables evenly around it.

4. Season both sides of the steak with the paprika, cumin, and garlic powder. Bake for 20 minutes.

5. Remove from the oven, cover with foil, and let rest for 10 minutes.

6. Divide the vegetables into 4 servings.

7. Slice the steak and divide evenly into 4 servings.

SUBSTITUTE! *To increase the fiber content in this dish, use diced sweet potatoes instead of the fingerling potatoes. To cut the calories, you can substitute cauliflower for the broccoli.*

STORAGE: *Store in the refrigerator for up to four days.*

Per serving: Calories: 282, Total Fat: 11g, Protein: 28g, Carbohydrates: 18g, Sugars: 4g, Fiber: 4g, Sodium: 87mg

MIXED BERRY CRISP

VEGETARIAN · VEGAN · NUT-FREE · DAIRY-FREE

This berry crisp skips the butter and uses less sugar than most. Even though it calls for sugar, the amount actually used for each serving is less than 1 tablespoon. While you want to use less added sugar to promote weight loss, having very small amounts occasionally is fine and won't derail your progress.

SERVES: *8*

PREP TIME: *10 minutes*

COOK TIME: *30 minutes*

Nonstick cooking spray

2 cups fresh blueberries

2 cups fresh raspberries

1 cup quartered
   fresh strawberries

2 tablespoons pure
   maple syrup

2 tablespoons cornstarch

1 cup old-fashioned
   rolled oats

¼ cup flour

1 teaspoon cinnamon

¼ cup brown sugar

½ cup unsweetened
   coconut flakes

1. Preheat the oven to 375°F. Spray a 9-by-9-inch glass baking pan with cooking spray.

2. Mix the berries together in the baking pan.

3. Stir the maple syrup and cornstarch together in a small bowl and pour over the fruit.

4. Combine the oats, flour, cinnamon, brown sugar, and coconut flakes in a medium bowl. Spread the mixture evenly over the fruit and bake for 30 minutes.

5. Divide into 8 servings.

SUBSTITUTE! *Use any kind of berry you prefer, as long as there are five cups of berries.*

STORAGE: *Store in the refrigerator for up to one week.*

SHORTCUT! *You can use frozen berries if fresh are not in season. When using frozen berries, increase the cooking time by 10 minutes.*

Per serving: Calories: 223, Total Fat: 9g, Protein: 4g, Carbohydrates: 33g, Sugars: 14g, Fiber: 7g, Sodium: 8mg

CHAPTER 9: NOTES

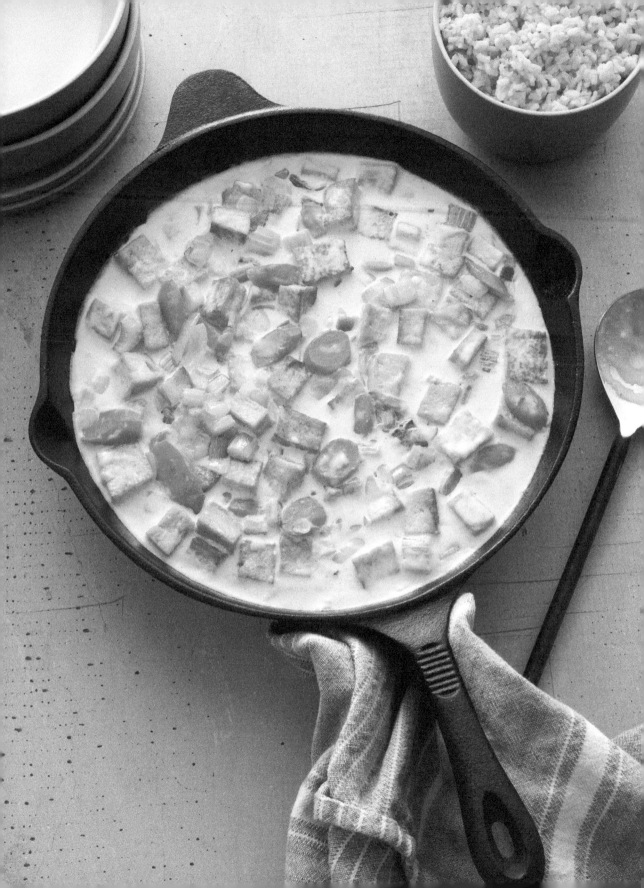

SKILLET

In each of the following recipes, double-check the recommended size and type of skillet. This often relates to capacity or whether you'll need to use a lid.

If oil is used in the cooking method, it may be divided between the protein and vegetables. This will be noted in the ingredients list.

Feel free to use frozen vegetables in place of fresh ones, but this may require an increase in cooking time to accommodate the temperature difference. In most cases, this should only amount to a 2- to 3-minute increase.

Tofu Curry,
p. 157

PAN-FRIED OATMEAL

VEGETARIAN • GLUTEN-FREE • NUT-FREE • 30 MINUTES OR LESS

Adding egg to oatmeal may seem unusual, but it's a great way to boost the protein in this traditional breakfast food and make it much more filling. Choose whatever fruit you have on hand to add. The combination of complex carbohydrates and protein also make this a great post-workout meal.

SERVES: *2*

PREP TIME: *5 minutes*

COOK TIME: *10 minutes*

2 teaspoons canola oil

¼ cup nonfat milk

¼ cup plain, fat-free Greek yogurt

1 egg

½ cup old-fashioned rolled oats

1 medium banana, sliced and divided

½ cup fresh or thawed frozen blueberries, divided

2 teaspoons pure maple syrup or honey, divided

1. In a small nonstick skillet, heat the canola oil over medium heat.

2. Pour the milk into a 2-cup measuring cup. Add the yogurt and stir with a fork.

3. Add the egg to the measuring cup and stir again to combine the mixture.

4. Add the oats to the skillet, stir to coat with the oil, and spread evenly over the bottom of the skillet.

5. Pour the egg mixture over the oats. Cook for 3 to 5 minutes, stirring occasionally to cook evenly.

6. Divide into two bowls and top each with half of the banana slices, ¼ cup of blueberries, and 1 teaspoon of maple syrup.

STORAGE: *Store in the refrigerator for up to two days.*

SHORTCUT! *To save time prepping breakfast for the week, double this recipe and store the leftovers. When doubling, use a 10-inch skillet.*

Per serving: Calories: 257, Total Fat: 9g, Protein: 9g, Carbohydrates: 39g, Sugars: 17g, Fiber: 4g, Sodium: 50mg

SWEET POTATOES WITH SAUSAGE AND EGGS

VEGETARIAN • NUT-FREE • DAIRY-FREE • 30 MINUTES OR LESS

Vegetarian sausage is a great option when you want that savory flavor without the unhealthy fat found in traditional breakfast sausages. If you can't find sausage crumbles, you can cut up a patty or use vegan crumbles, which mimic the look and texture of ground beef. Using frozen diced sweet potatoes cuts the time of peeling and cutting a sweet potato, but you'll need to increase the cook time by about 10 minutes to cook through.

SERVES: *4*

PREP TIME: *10 minutes*

COOK TIME: *15 minutes*

6 ounces vegetarian breakfast sausage, crumbled

1 (10-ounce) package sweet potato pieces

¼ cup chopped onions

1 teaspoon dried oregano

4 large eggs

1. In a cast-iron skillet or sauté pan with a lid, heat the sausage according to package directions.

2. Add the sweet potatoes, onions, and oregano. Cook over medium heat for 7 to 9 minutes, or until the sweet potatoes are heated through.

3. Using a spoon, make 4 wells in the potato-sausage mix.

4. Break one egg into each well.

5. Cover the skillet, reduce the heat to low, and cook the eggs for about 4 minutes, or until the egg yolk is cooked to your preference.

6. Divide into 4 servings.

SUBSTITUTE! *If you're looking to cut some calories, you can swap out the sweet potatoes for butternut squash, which has only about half the calories per cup as sweet potatoes.*

Per serving: Calories: 200, Total Fat: 8g, Protein: 11g, Carbohydrates: 20g, Sugars: 4g, Fiber: 3g, Sodium: 109mg

TOFU CURRY

VEGETARIAN · GLUTEN-FREE · NUT-FREE

Made from soybeans, tofu is one of the few plant-based sources of complete protein that has all the essential amino acids the body needs. Select extra-firm tofu, which has a similar consistency to cooked chicken. Once it's combined with the vegetables, broth, and curry powder, you'll never miss the chicken in this flavorful dish.

SERVES: *4*

PREP TIME: *35 minutes*

COOK TIME: *15 minutes*

16 ounces extra-firm tofu

1 cup nonfat milk, divided

1 tablespoon cornstarch

¾ cup low-sodium
  vegetable broth

Nonstick cooking spray

1 cup celery, diced

½ cup onions, diced

½ cup carrots, sliced

1 teaspoon jarred,
  minced garlic

2 teaspoons curry powder

Hot, cooked brown
  rice (optional)

1. To drain the tofu, wrap it in two layers of paper towels or a clean dish towel. Put the wrapped tofu on a plate, put a cutting board or another plate on top of it, and add an object such as a heavy can to compress the tofu and remove excess water. Let it drain for 30 minutes.

2. In a 2-cup measuring cup, mix together ¼ cup milk and the cornstarch until smooth. Add the remaining milk and the broth to the measuring cup and mix until smooth.

3. When the tofu is drained, cut it into ½-inch cubes.

4. Heat a 12-inch cast-iron skillet or sauté pan over medium heat. Spray with cooking spray and add the celery, onions, carrots, and garlic. Sauté for about 5 minutes, or until softened.

5. Add the tofu cubes to the vegetables and sauté for 3 to 4 minutes, or until the tofu is browned.

6. Stir the milk mixture and pour it into the skillet. Bring to a simmer, stir, and cook for 2 minutes.

7. Stir in the curry powder until it is evenly mixed into the tofu and vegetables.

8. Remove from the heat, divide into 4 servings, and serve with the rice (if using).

SHORTCUT! *Complete step 1 up to one day before, storing the tofu in the refrigerator as it drains. This will shorten the prep time to 15 minutes when preparing the dish.*

Per serving: Calories: 156, Total Fat: 7g, Protein: 14g, Carbohydrates: 12g, Sugars: 5g, Fiber: 2g, Sodium: 86mg

SHRIMP AND SQUASH SKILLET

GLUTEN-FREE • NUT-FREE • DAIRY-FREE • 30 MINUTES OR LESS

Summer squash come in a range that includes zucchini and yellow squash. Select any variety for this recipe. When cutting the squash, the slices should be the diameter of a silver dollar. If the squash is wider, cut the pieces into half-moons to allow for even cooking. Old Bay Seasoning is a blend of several herbs and spices and is sold in the spice aisle at the grocery store. The flavor of the shrimp and Old Bay will stand out from the mild-flavored squash.

SERVES: *4*

PREP TIME: *5 minutes*

COOK TIME: *10 minutes*

1 tablespoon olive oil

1 pound zucchini or yellow squash or a combination of both, sliced

1 red bell pepper, diced

2 garlic cloves, crushed, or 2 teaspoons jarred, minced garlic

1 pound raw medium shrimp, peeled

1 teaspoon Old Bay Seasoning or Cajun seasoning

Hot, cooked brown rice (optional)

1 lemon, quartered

1. In a 10-inch skillet, heat the oil over medium heat.

2. Add the squash, bell pepper, and garlic. Cook for about 5 minutes, or until softened.

3. Add the shrimp and toss with the vegetables. Cook for 2 to 3 minutes, or until the shrimp is fully cooked.

4. Add the Old Bay and toss to coat the shrimp and vegetables. Cook for 1 minute.

5. If serving with the rice, divide it into four plates or bowls and top with the shrimp and squash mixture.

6. Squeeze the juice of a lemon quarter over each.

STORAGE: *Store in the refrigerator for up to three days.*

SHORTCUT! *Buy raw shrimp already peeled to save time during prep.*

Per serving: Calories: 172, Total Fat: 5g, Protein: 26g, Carbohydrates: 8g, Sugars: 4g, Fiber: 2g, Sodium: 428mg

CHICKEN WITH BEANS AND GREENS

GLUTEN-FREE • NUT-FREE • DAIRY-FREE • 30 MINUTES OR LESS

Navy beans are white beans that are smaller than either Great Northern or cannellini beans. These three varieties can be used in recipes interchangeably without much difference in nutrition or flavor. Adding beans to a dish with chicken and kale boosts the protein and fiber content, both of which help with feeling full and eating less overall.

SERVES: *4*

PREP TIME: *10 minutes*

COOK TIME: *15 minutes*

2 cups low-sodium chicken broth

1 tablespoon chopped fresh rosemary

1 pound boneless, skinless chicken breast, cut into 1-inch pieces

2 (15-ounce) cans navy beans, drained and rinsed

10 ounces kale, chopped

½ teaspoon freshly ground black pepper

1. In a 10-inch cast-iron skillet or sauté pan, combine the broth and rosemary and bring to a simmer over medium heat.

2. Add the chicken and cook for 3 to 5 minutes.

3. Add the navy beans, kale, and pepper. Cook for about 4 minutes, or until the internal temperature of the chicken reaches 165°F.

4. Divide into 4 servings.

SUBSTITUTE! *Depending on what you have on hand, you can use spinach or collard greens in place of the kale.*

STORAGE: *Store in the refrigerator for up to four days or in the freezer for up to six months.*

SHORTCUT! *To save both prep and cooking time, you can use 3 cups precooked rotisserie chicken in place of the raw chicken. Skip to step 3, adding the chicken at the same time as the beans and kale.*

Per serving: Calories: 366, Total Fat: 4g, Protein: 39g, Carbohydrates: 44g, Sugars: 1g, Fiber: 16g, Sodium: 124mg

LEMON CHICKEN ORZO WITH ASPARAGUS

NUT-FREE • DAIRY-FREE

This colorful dish includes nearly every food group: tomato is a fruit; asparagus is a vegetable; orzo, which is a small pasta shaped like a grain of rice, is a grain; and chicken is protein. Recipes like this one help ensure that both your meal and overall diet are balanced.

SERVES: *4*

PREP TIME: *10 minutes*

COOK TIME: *25 minutes*

1 pound boneless, skinless chicken breasts

1 tablespoon olive oil

2 teaspoons lemon pepper, divided

2 cups low-sodium chicken broth

1 cup orzo

1 teaspoon dried oregano

1-pound fresh asparagus, cut into 1½- to 2-inch pieces

1 cup halved grape or cherry tomatoes

2 tablespoons lemon juice

1. Put the chicken breasts in a disposable zip-top bag, remove the air, and seal.

2. Using a meat mallet or rolling pin, pound or roll the chicken breasts into a thin layer.

3. In a 10-inch sauté pan, heat the oil over medium heat.

4. Place the chicken breasts in a single layer in the pan and season with 1 teaspoon lemon pepper. Cook on each side for about 2 minutes, adding the remaining lemon pepper after flipping the chicken.

5. Add the broth, orzo, and oregano. Cover and simmer for 8 to 10 minutes.

6. Add the asparagus and cook for 4 minutes.

7. Add the cherry tomatoes and lemon juice, stirring to blend.

8. Divide into 4 servings.

SUBSTITUTE! *Depending on what you have on hand, you can use pearl or Israeli couscous instead of orzo.*

STORAGE: *Store in the refrigerator for up to four days.*

SHORTCUT! *To save some time, you can use precut frozen asparagus instead of fresh asparagus.*

Per serving: Calories: 353, Total Fat: 6g, Protein: 35g, Carbohydrates: 40g, Sugars: 6g, Fiber: 5g, Sodium: 117mg

TURKEY STIR-FRY

NUT-FREE • DAIRY-FREE • 30 MINUTES OR LESS

The variety of frozen vegetables found in the freezer section of the grocery store is an easy shortcut for many dishes including a stir-fry. Stir-fry vegetables can include peppers, onions, snow peas, and water chestnuts, like in this recipe, or can be a different combination. Lean turkey breast, chicken broth, and Sriracha all provide a ton of flavor in this dish.

SERVES: 4

PREP TIME: *15 minutes*

COOK TIME: *15 minutes*

2 tablespoons olive oil, divided

1 pound turkey breast tenderloins or ground turkey breast

2 red bell peppers, sliced

1 medium yellow onion, sliced

½ cup snow peas, trimmed

1 (8-ounce) can sliced water chestnuts, drained

3 garlic cloves, minced, or 3 teaspoons jarred, minced garlic

½ cup low-sodium chicken broth

3 tablespoons low-sodium soy sauce

1 tablespoon Sriracha Hot Chili Sauce (optional)

1 tablespoon water (optional)

Hot, cooked rice (optional)

1. In a 10-inch sauté pan, heat 1 tablespoon of the oil over medium heat.

2. Add the turkey and cook for 5 to 6 minutes. The turkey does not need to be fully cooked through.

3. Add the remaining 1 tablespoon of oil to the pan and add the bell peppers, onion, snow peas, water chestnuts, and garlic. Sauté for 5 minutes.

4. In a 1- to 2-cup measuring cup, combine the broth, soy sauce, and Sriracha (if using). If not using Sriracha, add 1 tablespoon of water.

5. Pour the liquid over the turkey and vegetables, mixing to distribute the sauce evenly. Simmer for 2 minutes, or until the turkey reaches an internal temperature of 165°F.

6. Divide into 4 servings. Serve with the rice (if using).

SUBSTITUTE! *Depending on what you have on hand, use chicken breast tenderloin in place of the turkey breast tenderloin.*

STORAGE: *Store in the refrigerator for up to four days.*

SHORTCUT! *To save time slicing vegetables, use a 20-ounce bag of frozen stir-fry vegetables for the vegetables. Increase the cooking time by 5 minutes before adding the sauce.*

Per serving: Calories: 315, Total Fat: 9g, Protein: 32g, Carbohydrates: 30g, Sugars: 6g, Fiber: 2g, Sodium: 649mg

BEEF FAJITAS

NUT-FREE • 30 MINUTES OR LESS

Using smaller tortillas in this recipe decreases the overall portion size. If you use larger tortillas, such as 8 to 10 inches, use one tortilla per serving. If desired, skip the tortillas completely and make it a beef fajita bowl.

SERVES: *4*

PREP TIME: *10 minutes*

COOK TIME: *15 minutes*

1 pound flank steak, cut into thin strips

1 medium red bell pepper, sliced

1 medium green bell pepper, sliced

½ red onion, sliced

2 teaspoons chili powder

1 teaspoon paprika

1 teaspoon ground cumin

½ teaspoon salt

8 (6-inch) flour tortillas

½ cup shredded pepper Jack cheese, divided

1 medium avocado, cut into 8 pieces

1. Heat a cast-iron skillet over medium heat. When it is hot, sear the steak for 1 minute per side.

2. Add the bell peppers and onion. Sauté for 3 to 5 minutes.

3. Reduce the heat to low and add the chili powder, paprika, cumin, and salt, tossing to coat the vegetables and meat evenly.

4. Divide the meat and peppers evenly among the 8 tortillas.

5. Top each fajita with 1 tablespoon of cheese and 1 slice of avocado.

SUBSTITUTE! *For more variety, you can use chicken strips in place of the beef.*

STORAGE: *Store the meat and vegetable mixture in the refrigerator for up to four days.*

SHORTCUT! *To save time slicing the vegetables, use a 16- to 20-ounce package of frozen peppers and onion mix for the vegetables.*

Per serving: Calories: 546, Total Fat: 25g, Protein: 34g, Carbohydrates: 46g, Sugars: 5g, Fiber: 7g, Sodium: 741mg

CHEESEBURGER PASTA SKILLET

NUT-FREE

The taste of this one-skillet recipe mimics a cheeseburger. While it's not quite the same as the sandwich, lean ground beef gives it the familiar cheeseburger taste. Add the optional toppings of shredded lettuce and tomatoes to give it a cheeseburger feel.

SERVES: 4

PREP TIME: *10 minutes*

COOK TIME: *25 minutes*

1 pound 95 percent lean
  ground beef

½ cup chopped onions

½ teaspoon garlic powder

2 cups low-sodium
  beef broth

1 (15-ounce) can low-sodium
  tomato sauce

8 ounces whole wheat rotini
  or elbow pasta

½ cup shredded cheddar
  cheese, divided

1. In a 10-inch sauté pan with a lid, cook the ground beef, chopped onions, and garlic powder over medium heat for about 5 minutes, or until the meat is browned.

2. Drain the fat from the skillet.

3. Add the broth and tomato sauce, stirring to mix.

4. Add the pasta and stir to mix it well into the meat mixture.

5. Bring the mixture to a simmer, cover, and cook for 9 to 13 minutes, or until the pasta is fully cooked.

6. Divide into 4 servings and top each with 2 tablespoons of cheese.

SUBSTITUTE! *If you'd prefer to avoid red meat, you can substitute lean ground turkey breast for the ground beef.*

STORAGE: *Store in the refrigerator for up to four days.*

Per serving: Calories: 451, Total Fat: 12g, Protein: 38g, Carbohydrates: 48g, Sugars: 7g, Fiber: 8g, Sodium: 745mg

CARAMELIZED PINEAPPLE

VEGETARIAN • VEGAN • GLUTEN-FREE • NUT-FREE • DAIRY-FREE • 30 MINUTES OR LESS

Getting fresh pineapple without having to cut it up yourself is as easy as heading to the grocery store and looking for it in the produce aisle. This tropical fruit is a good source of potassium, vitamin C, and fiber. Eating pineapple plain is just fine, but you can turn it into a treat by heating it and adding more flavors. Eat this dish alone, add it to yogurt or oatmeal, or use it as a topping for frozen yogurt.

SERVES: *4*

PREP TIME: *5 minutes*

COOK TIME: *10 minutes*

10 ounces fresh
  pineapple spears

⅓ cup pure maple syrup

½ teaspoon cinnamon

2 tablespoons unsweetened
  shredded coconut

1. Heat a medium cast-iron or nonstick skillet over medium-high heat. Brown the pineapple spears in the skillet, turning to brown on all sides.

2. Pour the maple syrup over the pineapple and add the cinnamon, turning to evenly coat the fruit.

3. Remove from the heat and top with the coconut.

4. Divide into 4 servings.

SUBSTITUTE! *Depending on what you have on hand, you can substitute a 20-ounce can of 100 percent pineapple chunks or slices in its own juice, drained, for the fresh pineapple.*

STORAGE: *Store in the refrigerator for up to one week.*

Per serving: Calories: 147, Total Fat: 4g, Protein: 1g, Carbohydrates: 29g, Sugars: 23g, Fiber: 2g, Sodium: 6mg

CHAPTER 10: NOTES

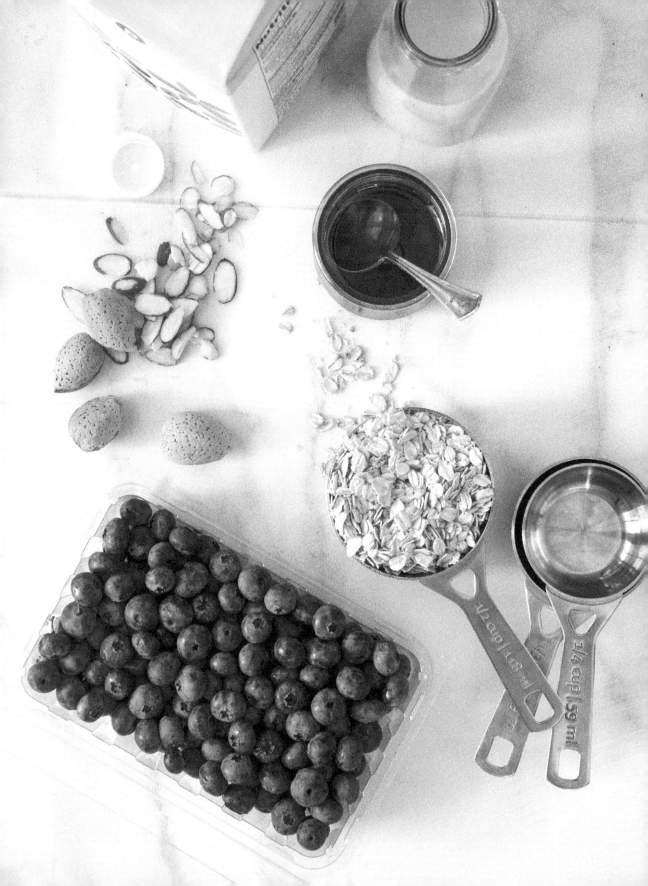

MEASUREMENT CONVERSIONS

Volume Equivalents (Liquid)

US Standard	US Standard (ounces)	Metric (approximate)
2 tablespoons	1 fl. oz.	30 mL
¼ cup	2 fl. oz.	60 mL
½ cup	4 fl. oz.	120 mL
1 cup	8 fl. oz.	240 mL
1½ cups	12 fl. oz.	355 mL
2 cups or 1 pint	16 fl. oz.	475 mL
4 cups or 1 quart	32 fl. oz.	1 L
1 gallon	128 fl. oz.	4 L

Oven Temperatures

Fahrenheit	Celsius (approximate)
250°F	120°C
300°F	150°C
325°F	165°C
350°F	180°C
375°F	190°C
400°F	200°C
425°F	220°C
450°F	230°C

Volume Equivalents (Dry)

US Standard	Metric (approximate)
⅛ teaspoon	0.5 mL
¼ teaspoon	1 mL
½ teaspoon	2 mL
¾ teaspoon	4 mL
1 teaspoon	5 mL
1 tablespoon	15 mL
¼ cup	59 mL
⅓ cup	79 mL
½ cup	118 mL
⅔ cup	156 mL
¾ cup	177 mL
1 cup	235 mL
2 cups or 1 pint	475 mL
3 cups	700 mL
4 cups or 1 quart	1 L

Weight Equivalents

US Standard	Metric (approximate)
½ ounce	15 g
1 ounce	30 g
2 ounces	60 g
4 ounces	115 g
8 ounces	225 g
12 ounces	340 g
16 ounces or 1 pound	455 g

REFERENCES

American Cancer Society. "American Cancer Society Guidelines on Nutrition and Physical Activity for Cancer Prevention." Accessed August 2, 2019. https://www.cancer.org/healthy/eat-healthy -get-active/acs-guidelines-nutrition-physical-activity-cancer-prevention/guidelines.html.

American Diabetes Association. "Making Healthy Food Choices." Accessed August 2, 2019. http://www.diabetes.org/food-and-fitness/food/what-can-i-eat/making-healthy-food-choices /?loc=ff-slabnav.

American Heart Association. "The American Heart Association Diet and Lifestyle Recommenda- tions." Accessed August 2, 2019. https://www.heart.org/en/healthy-living/healthy-eating/eat-smart /nutrition-basics/aha-diet-and-lifestyle-recommendations.

Hirotsu, Camila, Sergio Tufik, and Monica Levy Andersen. "Interactions between Sleep, Stress, and Metabolism: From Physiological to Pathological Conditions." *Sleep Science (São Paulo, Brazil)* 8, no. 3 (November 2015): 143-52. doi:10.1016/j.slsci.2015.09.002.

Institute of Medicine (U.S.) Committee on Diet and Health, Woteki CE, and Thomas PR. *Eat for Life: The Food and Nutrition Board's Guide to Reducing Your Risk of Chronic Disease*. Washington, D.C.: National Academies Press (U.S.); 1992. Chapter 7, "Protein, Carbohydrates, And Chronic Diseases." Available from: https://www.ncbi.nlm.nih.gov/books/NBK235012/.

National Sleep Foundation. "What Temperature Should Your Bedroom Be?" Accessed August 2, 2019. https://www.sleepfoundation.org/bedroom-environment/touch/what-temperature-should -your-bedroom-be.

Neff, Roni A., Danielle Edwards, Anne Palmer, Rebecca Ramsing, Allison Righter, and Julia Wolfson. "Reducing Meat Consumption in the USA: A Nationally Representative Survey of Attitudes and Behaviours." *Public Health Nutrition* 21, no. 10 (July 2018): 1835–44. doi:10.1017 /S1368980017004190.

Safe Fruits and Veggies. "Pesticide Residue Calculator." Accessed August 2, 2019. https://www.safe fruitsandveggies.com/pesticide-residue-calculator/.

Thoma, Myriam V., Roberto La Marca, Rebecca Bronnimann, Linda Finkel, Ulrike Ehlert, and Urs M. Nater. "The Effect of Music on the Human Stress Response." *PLOS One* 8, no. 8 (August 2013): e70156. doi:10.1371/journal.pone.0070156.

Warburton, Darren E. R., Crystal Whitney Nicol, and Shannon S. D. Bredin. "Health Benefits of Physi- cal Activity: The Evidence." *CMAJ* 174, no. 6 (March 2006): 801–9. doi:10.1503/cmaj.051351.

World Health Organization. "Healthy Diet." Accessed August 2, 2019. https://www.who.int /en/news-room/fact-sheets/detail/healthy-diet.

INDEX

ACKNOWLEDGMENTS

I would like to acknowledge and thank my friends and family for their contributions and support that led to this book:

Neily, for the videos we did in Charleston with Take-Two in Philly; Barbra, for the guidance that said to write a book; Yvonne, for being a writing/accountability partner; Karen, for the cheers, support, and daily gratitudes; Carrie, for loaning me that appliance so I wouldn't have to add more clutter; Ted, who said all the trial recipes tasted good even when they didn't; and my employees Max, security detail, and Blue, customer service, who mostly sleep on the job but also help with kitchen cleanup.

ABOUT THE AUTHOR

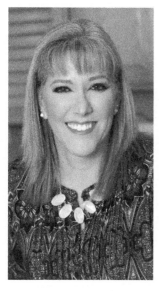

SHELLEY RAEL, MS, RDN, is a registered dietitian nutritionist who was thrilled to find out that she could have a career that was all about thinking and talking about food. She helps people change their mind-set about food, eliminating rules, and judgment while supporting a lifestyle that helps people with food acceptance, eating food they love, and still being able to lose weight through one-on-one and group programs. Rather than gimmicks, supplements, or fad diets, Shelley works with individuals to find what works for them and helps them create action plans so that they can lose weight for good year-round. Fads, trends, and quick fixes will come and go, but eating will always be necessary. Shelley is a wife to one husband, mother to one son, nana to one granddaughter, and mom to two rescue dogs in New Mexico.